STATISTICS *for*
HEALTH CARE RESEARCH

A Practical Workbook

STATISTICS *for*
HEALTH CARE RESEARCH

A Practical Workbook

Susan K. Grove, PhD, APRN, BC, ANP, GNP
Associate Dean and Graduate Advisor
School of Nursing
The University of Texas at Arlington
Arlington, Texas

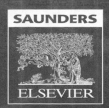

SAUNDERS

ELSEVIER

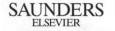

11830 Westline Industrial Drive
St. Louis, Missouri 63146

STATISTICS FOR HEALTH CARE RESEARCH: ISBN: 978-1-4160-0226-0
A PRACTICAL WORKBOOK
Copyright © 2007 by Saunders, an imprint of Elsevier Inc.

Notice

ISBN: 978-1-4160-0226-0

Acquisitions Editor: Barbara Cullen
Developmental Editor: Jacqueline Twomey
Publishing Services Manager: Jeff Patterson
Design Direction: Jyotika Shroff

Printed in the United States of America

Last digit is the print number: 9   8   7   6   5   4   3   2   1

To my husband:
Jay Suggs for his constant encouragement

and

To our future:
Monece, Steve, and Baby Jack Appleton
Samantha Nicole Suggs and Scott Horn

CONTRIBUTORS

Aneta Grodzensky, MSN, ANP
Nurse Practitioner
Rockford Radiology Associates
Rockford, Illinois

Sheila Harzman, MSN, RN, CPNP
Pediatric Nurse Practitioner
Medical & Surgical Clinic of Irving
Irving, Texas

Judy LeFlore, PhD, MSN, MS, RNC, NNP, CPNP-AC, CPNP-PC
Director, Pediatric and Acute Care Pediatric Nurse Practitioner Programs
The University of Texas at Arlington
Arlington, Texas

Amy Morse, MSN
Pediatric Nurse Practitioner Student
University of Texas at Arlington
Arlington, Texas

Gena Nelson, MSN, BS, RN, GPMHNP
Nurse Practitioner
Holiner Psychiatric Group
Dallas, Texas

Amanda L. Shaw, MSN, RN, CPNP
Pediatric Nurse Practitioner
Pediatric Health Center at Presbyterian Hospital of Dallas
Dallas, Texas

Rhoda Watson, MSN, BS Elem Ed, RN, ACNP
Instructor, Division of Gastroenterology
University of North Texas Health Science Center;
Physicians Surgical Center of Fort Worth;
Plaza Medical Center of Fort Worth;
JPS Health Network
Fort Worth, Texas

REVIEWERS

Gregory A. Bechtel, PhD, MPH
Professor, School of Nursing
University of North Carolina Wilmington
Wilmington, North Carolina

Gina S. Brown, PhD, RN
Dean, School of Graduate and Professional
  Studies
Columbia Union College
Takoma Park, Maryland

Ronald M. Dick, PhD, RPh
Professor of Anesthesiology
Barry University
Miami Shores, Florida

Bryan W. Griffin, PhD
Associate Professor
Department of Curriculum, Foundations, and
  Research
Georgia Southern University
Statesboro, Georgia

Anne Cowley Herzog, MSN, RN
Professor of Nursing
Cypress College
Cypress, California

Barbara J. Hoerst, PhD, RN
Assistant Professor
LaSalle University School of Nursing
Philadelphia, Pennsylvania

Janet T. Ihlenfeld†, PhD, RN
Professor, Department of Nursing
D'Youville College
Buffalo, New York

Jean Jacko, PhD, RN
Associate Professor, School of Nursing
Capital University
Columbus, Ohio

Angela M. McNelis, PhD, RN
Assistant Professor
Indiana University School of Nursing
Indianapolis, Indiana

Barbara Napoli, MBA, BA
Our Lady of the Lake College
Baton Rouge, Louisiana

Chris Seckman, MSN, RN
Associate Professor
Clarkson College
Omaha, Nebraska

Pam Springer, PhD, MSN
Professor and Department Chair
Department of Nursing
College of Health Sciences
Boise State University
Boise, Idaho

Susan K. Steele, DNS, RN, AOCN
Assistant Professor, School of Nursing
Louisiana State University Health Sciences
  Center
New Orleans, Louisiana

Georgianna M. Thomas, EdD, MSN, RN
Dean of Nursing
West Suburban College of Nursing
Oak Park, Illinois

Joan Tilghman, PhD, RN, APRN-BC
Associate Dean of Masters Education
Helene Fuld School of Nursing
Coppin State University
Baltimore, Maryland

Golden Tradewell, PhD, RN
Chair, Department of Nursing
Southern Arkansas University
Magnolia, Arkansas

Michael B. Worrell, PhD
Assistant Professor of Biology
Hanover College
Hanover, Indiana

†Deceased.

PREFACE

With the emphasis in health care today on evidence-based practice, it is more important than ever for health care professionals to understand essential information about measurement, sampling, and statistical analysis techniques. Having this background enables us to read and understand research results, and to know if, when, and how those results should be used to provide evidence-based care to patients and families.

Statistics for Health Care Research provides a hands-on approach to understanding levels of measurement, measurement reliability and validity, nonprobability and probability sampling methods, and common statistical analysis techniques. It allows the reader to first read about an analysis technique, and then apply this knowledge to a published health care study. The workbook starts by establishing a basic understanding of levels of measurement and progresses to more complicated statistical analysis techniques.

The workbook is organized into 45 exercises, which are focused on measurement, sampling, or statistical techniques. Each exercise provides the content needed to address the topic of the exercise—be it nominal level of measurement or multiple regression—and includes the following sections:

- ▣ Statistical Technique in Review
- ▣ Research Article
- ▣ Study Questions
- ▣ Answers to Study Questions
- ▣ Questions to be Graded

The *Statistical Technique in Review* at the beginning of each exercise provides a brief summary of the featured technique. The *Research Article* section then provides a bibliographic reference to a pertinent published study from the health sciences literature. An *Introduction* follows to provide the reader with a base from which to interpret the study. A section called *Relevant Study Results,* based on the cited article, provides a relevant example taken directly from a current, published health sciences study. The *Study Questions* section guides the reader in examining the statistical technique in the research article. The *Answers to Study Questions* section provides immediate feedback to ensure content mastery or identify areas needing further study. Finally, *Questions to Be Graded* are provided at the end of each exercise; these questions can be submitted to the instructor for additional feedback. (Pages are perforated for easy removal.)

Statistics for Health Care Research was developed to meet the need for a statistics workbook specifically focused on *health care* research. It is therefore based on high-quality research articles from the health sciences literature rather than the social sciences literature.

Useful at both the undergraduate and graduate level, *Statistics for Health Care Research* offers not only a practical review of the most commonly used statistical analysis techniques but also a realistic context in which to learn each technique. By reviewing each technique in the context of relevant health sciences literature, the student can become familiar with analyzing actual study results rather than performing statistical calculations in isolation. The workbook is equally valuable for the practicing clinician because each exercise provides a concise review of a statistical technique that health care professionals need to understand. It is my hope that the statistical exercises that introduce students and clinicians to current health sciences research literature will also help to expand their desire for using research findings in clinical practice.

EVOLVE LEARNING RESOURCES

Resources for both students and instructors are provided on an Evolve Learning Resources website at http://evolve.elsevier.com/Grove/statistics/. For students and instructors, links are provided to all of the source articles used in the workbook. For instructors, an Answer Key for the *Questions to Be Graded* is provided to help ensure that students have mastered the content.

ACKNOWLEDGMENTS

I would like to express my great appreciation to the contributors to this text: Dr. Judy LeFlore, Sheila Harzman, Aneta Grodzensky, Amy Morse, Gena Nelson, Amanda Shaw, and Rhoda Watson. It was my pleasure to work with each of you and to have the opportunity to expand our understanding of statistical knowledge together.

Special thanks are extended to Bryan Griffin, whose statistical knowledge was invaluable to me in ensuring the quality and accuracy of the information in this workbook. I also want to thank both Bryan Griffin and Barbara Napoli for their painstaking reviews and for helping me to ensure the accuracy and clarity of the content at every step. I appreciate the time and effort that they spent verifying that this text is as accurate and relevant as possible. Any errors that remain are, of course, my own. I would also like to recognize our team of reviewers for their guidance in the development of this workbook.

Finally, I would like to thank the people at Elsevier who worked tirelessly to produce this book: Lee Henderson, Senior Editor; Maureen Iannuzzi, Senior Developmental Editor; Jacqueline Twomey, Editorial Assistant; Jeanne Genz, Project Manager; and Amy Shehi, Multimedia Producer.

Susan K. Grove

CONTENTS

1

IDENTIFYING LEVEL OF MEASUREMENT: NOMINAL

STATISTICAL TECHNIQUE IN REVIEW

The levels of measurement were identified in 1946 by Stevens, who organized the rules for assigning numbers to objects so that a hierarchy of measurement was established. The measurement levels, from lowest to highest level, are nominal, ordinal, interval, and ratio. The higher the level of measurement achieved in a study, the stronger the data analysis technique that can be used to analyze the data. Variables measured at the **nominal level of measurement** are at the lowest level and must follow three rules: (1) the data categories must be exhaustive (each datum will fit into at least one category identified by the researcher), (2) the data categories must be exclusive (each datum will fit into only one category), and (3) the data cannot be rank ordered (Burns & Grove, 2007). Nominal data differ from ordinal data in that ordinal data can be rank ordered. Examples of nominal data include gender, ethnicity, marital status, medical diagnoses, and primary language.

Nonparametric or distribution-free analysis techniques can be used to analyze nominal level data to describe variables, examine relationships among variables, and determine differences between groups in distribution-free or non-normally distributed samples. The assumptions of nonparametric statistics are: (1) values from measurement of study variables need not be normally distributed in the sample, and (2) the level of measurement of study variables is usually nominal or ordinal. The mode is the only measure of central tendency that can be calculated for nominal data and is the most frequent occurring value in a data set (see Exercise 15). Frequencies and percentages are also used to analyze nominal data to describe the study or demographic variables (see Exercises 4, 5, and 6). Chi square is an analysis technique conducted on nominal data to identify relationships and differences in studies (see Exercises 40 and 41).

RESEARCH ARTICLE

Source: Cuellar, N., Cochran, S., Ladner, C., Mercier, B., Townsend, A., Harbaugh, B., et al. (2003). Depression and the use of conventional and nonconventional interventions by rural patients. *Journal of the American Psychiatric Nurses Association, 9*(5), 151–8.

Introduction

In their study Cuellar and colleagues (2003) examined four groups of individuals with different health issues in rural areas to determine if they were depressed. They also identified and compared the conventional and nonconventional interventions that were implemented for depression in the four groups. The four groups studied were patients with breast cancer, patients with myocardial infarction (MI), patients with stroke, and care providers. In this comparative descriptive study, 120 participants completed the Center for Epidemiologic Studies Depression Index (CES-D). The results of the study showed that 37% of the patients were depressed and that only 13 of the 44 individuals were being treated with antidepressants. The researchers also found that 73% of the married participants were depressed and those who were unemployed or retired were more likely to be depressed than those who were employed. There were no significant differences among the four groups in the effectiveness of the types of treatments they received for depression. The researchers encouraged health care providers to screen and treat depression, "especially in rural areas where poverty, isolation, and lack of mental health services are common" (Cuellar et al., 2003, p. 151).

Relevant Study Results

The researchers indicated that when depression occurs with comorbid medical conditions, it can lead to underdiagnosis and undertreatment in these types of patients. In rural areas, patients may have less access to mental health care and experience a greater stigma for mental health problems. Thus, a comprehensive history and physical exam are important during assessment of patients with comorbid medical conditions in order to screen for depression. The subjects were asked to participate by nurses at the health centers where they received care. Researchers interviewed the subjects and observed them for emotional changes during the interview process. When the groups were compared, the researchers found no significant difference in the amount of depression between the four groups. However, they did find that females were more depressed than males; patients with MIs had the least evidence of physical symptomology; and patients who had suffered a stroke had the highest mean scores for depressive symptomology. The demographic data for the subjects are presented in Table 1, and the range of scores for the subjects on the CES-D Index is presented in Table 2 (Cuellar et al., 2003).

TABLE 1 ■ Frequency Counts and Percentages on Demographic Data (N=120)		
Descriptive Variable	Total Sample: n (%)	Depressed ($n = 44$)
AGE (y)		
29–38	3 (2.5%)	0
39–48	16 (13.3%)	8 (18.2%)
49–58	35 (29.2%)	13 (29.5%)
59–68	37 (30.8%)	10 (22.7%)
69+	29 (24.2%)	13 (29.5%)
GENDER		
Male	45 (37.5%)	17 (38.6%)
Female	75 (62.5%)	27 (61.4%)
ETHNICITY		
Caucasian	97 (80.8%)	36 (81.8%)
African American	22 (18.3%)	7 (15.9%)
Asian	1 (.8%)	1 (2.3%)
MARITAL STATUS*		
Single	7 (6%)	0(0%)
Married	80 (67%)	32 (73%)
Divorced	11 (9%)	4 (9%)
Widowed	22 (18%)	8 (18%)
SOCIOECONOMIC STATUS		
Less than $20,000	54 (45.8%)	22 (51.2%)
$21–$40,000	40 (33.9%)	11 (25.6%)
$41–$60,000	13 (11%)	5 (11.6%)
$61–$80,000	7 (5.9%)	3 (7%)
More than $80,000	4 (3.3%)	2 (4.6%)
EMPLOYMENT STATUS*		
Employed	38 (31.7%)	6 (13.6%)
Unemployed	19 (15.8%)	13 (29.5%)
Retired	63 (52.5%)	25 (56.8%)

Note. *Using Chi Square analysis, significant at $p < .05$.

Cuellar, N., Cochran, S., Ladner, C., Mercier, B., Townsend, A., Harbaugh, B., et al. (2003). Depression and the use of conventional and nonconventional interventions by rural patients. *Journal of the American Psychiatric Nurses Association, 9*(5), p.155.

TABLE 2 ■ Frequency Counts and Percentages on Center for Epidemiologic Studies Depression Index (CES-D) Scores

Range of Scores	Total: N = 120	Percentage (%)
0–15 (not depressed)	76	63
16–20 (mild depression)	15	12.5
21–30 (moderate depression)	15	12.5
≥ 31 (severe depression)	14	12

Cuellar, N., Cochran, S., Ladner, C., Mercier, B., Townsend, A., Harbaugh, B., et al. (2003). Depression and the use of conventional and nonconventional interventions by rural patients. *Journal of the American Psychiatric Nurses Association, 9*(5), p. 155.

■ STUDY QUESTIONS

1. Identify the variables that are measured at the nominal level in Table 1.

2. Is age measured at the nominal level? Provide a rationale for your answer.

3. What is the mode for marital status in the total sample and in the depressed group?

4. How many of the depressed persons were unemployed? Would you have expected this finding? Provide a rationale for your answer.

5. How many of the depressed persons were married? Would you have expected this finding? Provide a rationale for your answer.

6. No depression was reported in the 29 to 38 age group. What are the possible reasons for this?

7. How many subjects and what percentage of the total sample were 49 years of age or older? Round your answer to the nearest tenth of a percent (%).

8. Nominal data categories should be exhaustive. In looking at Ethnicity in Table 1, are these ethnic categories exhaustive? Provide a rationale for your answer.

9. For which variables in this table can a median be calculated? What does this tell us about the level of measurement of the variables?

10. Are parametric or nonparametric statistical analysis techniques used to analyze nominal level data? Provide a rationale for your answer.

■ ANSWERS TO STUDY QUESTIONS

1. In Table 1, gender, ethnicity, marital status, and employment status were measured at the nominal level.

2. No, the age categories can be rank ordered and are therefore an example of ordinal level of measurement and not nominal level of measurement.

3. The mode for marital status is married with a frequency of 80 subjects, which was 67% of the total sample. The mode for the depressed group was also married with a frequency of 32, which was 73% of the depressed group.

4. 13 (29.5%) of the depressed persons were unemployed. Yes, you would expect that persons who have a comorbid condition and are experiencing depression might have a higher unemployment rate. In addition, unemployment might also lead to or increase depression. The evidence-based information on assessment, diagnosis, and management of depression is available online at http://www.guideline.gov.

5. 32 (73%) of the depressed persons were married. This is a higher number than might be expected. This finding is contradictory to other studies on depression, which have found that persons who are in an intact marriage are less depressed than people who are divorced or single (http://www.ahcpr.gov). However, these subjects have comorbid conditions (cancer, MI, or stroke) or are caregivers, which might explain the number of married subjects with depression.

6. One possible reason is that there are only 3 persons in that group and the number of subjects is too small to determine the incidence of depression for that age group. It should also be noted that the sample included subjects who were caregivers, stroke survivors, breast cancer survivors, and MI survivors, who are often older. The majority of the subjects were 49 and older.

7. 101 subjects or 84.2% of the sample were 49 years of age or older. Add $35 + 37 + 29 = 101$. Percent is found by $101 \div 120 = 0.8417 \times 100 = 84.2\%$. Or the percentages in Table 1 can be added together: $29.2\% + 30.8\% + 24.2\% = 84.2\%$.

8. Yes, for this sample the ethnic categories are exhaustive because all 120 subjects fit into one of the ethnic categories of Caucasian, African American, or Asian. However, for another study, these three ethnic categories might not cover all of the different ethnic backgrounds of those subjects participating in the study.

9. A median or middle score can be calculated for age and socioeconomic status, which means these variables are measured at the ordinal level. Since the variables are measured at the ordinal level, the categories can be rank ordered so that a middle score can be determined. The other variables are at the nominal level of measurement since they cannot be rank ordered.

10. Nonparametric statistical analysis techniques are used to analyze nominal and ordinal level data. Nominal data can only be sorted into categories that are mutually exclusive and exhaustive and nonparametric analyses can be conducted on this level of data. Parametric analyses are usually conducted on variables that are measured at the interval or ratio level.

■ EXERCISE 1   Questions to be Graded

1. What variable is presented in Table 2? What is the level of measurement of this variable? Provide a rationale for your answer.

2. How many subjects and what percentage of this sample had a CES-D score of 16 or higher?

3. What is the mode for employment status of the total sample and the depressed groups? Is this what you might expect for this sample?

4. Which ethnic group had the most individuals who are depressed?

5. What number and percentage of the 44 depressed subjects were treated with antidepressant medications? Do you think an adequate number received treatment with medication? Provide a rationale for your answer.

6. The researchers found that two of the participants used herbs and one used alternative therapies. Would you expect more or less use of herbs and alternative therapies in rural areas? Provide a rationale for your answer.

7. The researchers excluded persons from the study who had a history of psychiatric illness. Provide a rationale for excluding these persons.

8. In the Employment Status categories in Table 1, are the categories exhaustive for the total sample? Provide a rationale for your answer.

9. The article states that 1 out of 10 people in the United States suffer from depression. How do the results of this study compare to this figure? How might you explain any differences?

10. How are the results from this study useful in practice?

IDENTIFYING LEVEL OF MEASUREMENT: ORDINAL

STATISTICAL TECHNIQUE IN REVIEW

The levels of measurement from the lowest to the highest level are nominal, ordinal, interval, and ratio. **Ordinal level measurement** includes categories that can be rank ordered and also, like nominal level measurement, the categories are mutually exclusive and exhaustive (see Exercise 1). In ranking categories of a variable, each category must be recognized as higher or lower or better or worse than another category (Burns & Grove, 2007). However, with ordinal level of measurement, you do not know exactly how much higher or lower one subject's score is in relation to another subject's score on a variable . Thus, variables measured at the ordinal level do not have a continuum of values with equal distances between them as do variables measured at the interval level. For example, you could have subjects identify their levels of acute pain as "no pain," "mild pain," "moderate pain," or "severe pain." This is an example of ordinal level measurement of variable pain because the categories can be ranked from a low of "no pain" to a high of "severe pain." Even though the subjects' levels of pain can be ranked, you do not know the difference between the levels of pain. The difference between "no pain" and "mild pain" might be less than that between "moderate pain" and "severe pain." Thus, ordinal level data have unknown, unequal intervals between the categories, such as between the levels of pain.

Nonparametric statistical analysis techniques are used to analyze nominal and ordinal level data to describe variables, examine relationships among variables, and determine differences between groups in distribution-free samples. Descriptive statistical analyses such as median, range, frequency, percentage, and mode can be performed on ordinal level data (Burns & Grove, 2005). Spearman Rank-Order Correlation Coefficient is used to examine relationships among variables measured at the ordinal level (see Exercise 42). Mann-Whitney *U* Test and Wilcoxon Matched-Pairs Signed-Ranks Test can be used to determine differences between groups when study data are measured at the ordinal level (see Exercises 43 and 44).

RESEARCH ARTICLE

Source: Kuster, P. A., Badr, L. K., Chang, B. L., Wuerker, A. K., & Benjamin, A. E., (2004). Factors influencing health promoting activities of mothers caring for ventilator-assisted children. *Journal of Pediatric Nursing, 19*(4), 276-87.

Introduction

Kuster, Badr, Chang, Wuerker, and Benjamin (2004) conducted a descriptive correlational study to examine "the relationships among the functional status of the [ventilator-assisted] child, the impact of the illness on the family, coping, social support, and health-promotion activities of mothers who care for ventilator-assisted children at home" (Kuster et al., 2004, p. 276). The study included 38 mothers of ventilator-assisted children. Data collection occurred over a six-month period. The results of the study indicated that mothers' participation in health-promotion activities was related to the functional status of the child, impact on the family, and coping. Nurses are needed to assist mothers in coping and finding resources to manage the care of their child so that they can maintain their own health.

Relevant Study Results

The characteristics of the mothers of ventilator-assisted children (*N* = 38) are presented in Table 1. "There were 34 biological mothers, 2 adoptive mothers, 1 grandmother, and 1 foster mother in the sample. The mean age of the subjects was 37.5 years (*SD* = 9.77), and their ages ranged from 22 to 62 years of age. The majority of subjects (76.3%) were married, and over half (57.9%) described their employment status as 'homemaker.' The subjects were predominantly White/Non-Hispanic (42.1%) and Hispanic/Latina (36.8%). Five (13.2%) of the mothers completed the self-report questionnaire and interview in Spanish" (Kuster et al., 2004, p. 279).

TABLE 1 ■ Characteristics of the Mothers of Ventilator-Assisted Children (*N* = 38)		
Demographic Variables	Frequency	Percentage
MARITAL STATUS		
Single	2	5.3%
Married	29	76.3%
Separated	3	7.9%
Divorced	2	5.3%
Living Together	2	5.3%
ETHNICITY		
White/Non-Hispanic	16	42.1%
African American	3	7.9%
Hispanic/Latina	14	36.8%
Asian American	4	10.5%
Other	1	2.6%
EMPLOYMENT STATUS		
Employed Full-time	7	18.4%
Employed Part-time	4	10.5%
Unemployed/Not seeking	4	10.5%
Homemaker	22	57.9%
Other	1	2.6%
EDUCATION (HIGHEST LEVEL)		
4-Year College and Higher	7	18.5%
2-Year College	5	13.2%
Partial College	10	26.3%
High School Graduate/GED	10	26.3%
Junior High/Partial High School	4	10.5%
Under 7 years	2	5.3%
ESTIMATED YEARLY FAMILY INCOME		
Less than $5000	3	7.9%
$10,000–$19,999	7	18.4%
$20,000–$39,999	12	31.6%
$40,000–$59,999	4	10.5%
Greater than $60,000	12	31.6%

Kuster, P. A., Badr, L. K., Chang, B. L., Wuerker, A. K., & Benjamin, A. E., (2004). Factors influencing health promoting activities of mothers caring for ventilator-assisted children. *Journal of Pediatric Nursing, 19*(4), p. 279.

■ STUDY QUESTIONS

1. What level of measurement is the variable Marital Status? Provide a rationale for your response.

2. What level of measurement is the variable Estimated Yearly Family Income? Provide a rationale for your response.

3. Are the categories of Estimated Yearly Family Income exclusive and exhaustive? Provide a rationale for your answer.

4. Which category or categories of Estimated Yearly Family Income included the largest percentage (%) of mothers?

5. How many women had two years of college?

6. What level of measurement is the variable Ethnicity? Provide a rationale for your answer.

7. What level of measurement is the variable Educational Level? Provide a rationale for your response.

8. Is Employment Status measured at the ordinal level? Provide a rationale for your response.

9. Should the variable Employment Status be analyzed with parametric or nonparametric statistical analysis techniques? Provide a rationale for your answer.

■ ANSWERS TO STUDY QUESTIONS

1. The Marital Status variable is measured at the nominal level. The categories are single, married, separated, divorced, and living together, which are mutually exclusive and exhaustive. However, these categories cannot be ranked. Thus, this variable is measured at the nominal level and not the ordinal level.

2. The Estimated Yearly Family Income variable is measured at the ordinal level. The categories are less than $5,000, $10,000–$19,999, $20,000–$39,999, $40,000–$59,999, and greater than $60,000. These income categories can be rank ordered from the lowest to highest income levels. Thus the income variable is measured at the ordinal level.

3. The Estimated Yearly Family Income variable has exclusive and exhaustive categories. A subject could only mark one income level and all 38 subjects were identified with an income category so the categories were exhaustive. It appears as though the income category of $5,000–$9,999 is missing but since there was no subject that fell within that income range, it was not included.

4. The largest percentage of mothers falls into two estimated yearly family income categories of $20,000–$39,999 and greater than $60,000. There were 12 (31.6%) mothers in each of these two income categories.

5. Five women had two years of college.

6. The variable Ethnicity is measured at the nominal level because it includes mutually exclusive and exhaustive categories. These categories are White/Non-Hispanic, African American, Hispanic/Latina, Asian American, and other. The categories are exclusive because a subject could mark one category only, and the other category makes the categories exhaustive. However, the categories cannot be rank ordered, so ethnicity is measured at the nominal, not ordinal, level.

7. The variable Education level is measured at the ordinal level since the categories are exclusive, exhaustive, and can be ranked from higher level of education to lower level of education.

8. No. The Employment level variable is not measured at the ordinal level. The categories of employment cannot be rank ordered. Thus, the Employment level variable is measured at the nominal level.

9. The Employment level variable is measured at the nominal level. Data at the nominal level of measurement are usually analyzed with nonparametric statistics.

■ EXERCISE 2   Questions to be Graded

1. What demographic variables were measured at the nominal level of measurement? Provide a rationale for your answer.

2. What statistics were used to describe the demographic variable Estimated Yearly Family Income in this study? Were these appropriate?

3. Could additional descriptive statistics be conducted on the data for Estimated Yearly Family Income? Provide a rationale for your response.

4. Were the categories for the demographic variable Education (highest level) mutually exclusive, exhaustive, and rank ordered? Provide a rationale for your answer.

5. Can marital status be rank ordered? Provide a rationale for your answer.

6. Most women had what level of education? How would you interpret this result?

7. Should the demographic variable Educational level be analyzed with parametric or nonparametric statistical analysis techniques? Provide a rationale for your answer.

8. Could a median be determined for the education level data? If so, what would the median be for education in this study?

9. Are the intervals between the Estimated Yearly Family Income categories equal? Provide a rationale for your answer.

10. What number and percentage of women had an income less than $40,000? What does this result indicate?

IDENTIFYING LEVEL OF MEASUREMENT: INTERVAL/RATIO

STATISTICAL TECHNIQUE IN REVIEW

The levels of measurement were identified in 1946 by Stevens, who organized the rules for assigning numbers to objects so that a hierarchy of measurement was established. The measurement levels, from lowest to highest level, are nominal, ordinal, interval, and ratio. The higher the level of measurement achieved in a study, the stronger the data analysis technique that can be used to analyze the data. With **interval level of measurement,** the distances between intervals of the scale are numerically equal. However, with the interval scale, there is no absolute zero point at which the property being measured is absent. Examples of interval scales include Fahrenheit and Celsius temperature scales (Burns & Grove, 2007).

Ratio level of measurement is the highest form of measurement that adheres to the same rules as interval level measurements with numerically equal intervals on the scale. In addition, ratio level measurement has an absolute zero point, where at zero the property is absent, such as zero weight means absence of weight. Examples of variables that can be measured at the ratio level include weight, height, blood pressure, pulse, respiration, and laboratory values (Burns & Grove, 2007).

Statistics are divided into parametric and nonparametric categories. Nonparametric or distribution-free analysis techniques are typically used to analyze nominal and ordinal level data to describe variables, examine relationships among variables, and determine differences between groups. **Parametric statistics** are often used to analyze interval and ratio level data. The assumptions of parametric statistics include: (1) the distribution of scores in a sample are expected to be normal or approximately normal, (2) the level of measurement of variables is usually at least at the interval level, and (3) the data can be treated as obtained from a random sample (Burns & Grove, 2007). Parametric analyses are usually conducted on interval and ratio levels of data to describe variables, examine relationships among variables, and determine differences between groups. For example, means and standard deviations can be conducted to describe variables, measured at the interval or ratio level (see Exercise 16). Pearson's Product-Moment Correlation Coefficient (see Exercise 23) is used to determine significant relationships between variables, and the *t*-test (see Exercise 29) is conducted to determine significant differences between groups. **Significant results** are those in keeping with the outcomes predicted by the researcher, where the null hypothesis is rejected. Significant results are usually identified by * or p values $\leq$ alpha (α), which is often set at 0.05 for a study. So any p values ≤ 0.05 are considered significant. Since the analysis techniques are similar for variables measured at the interval and ratio levels, the levels of measurement will frequently be referred to as interval/ratio without differentiating between the two levels in this text.

RESEARCH ARTICLE

Source: Fallis, W. M. (2005). The effect of urine flow rate on urinary bladder temperature in critically ill adults. *Heart & Lung, 34*(3), 209-16.

Introduction

The researcher of this study set out to determine the effect of urine flow rate on bladder temperature as well as the relationship between urinary bladder temperature and pulmonary artery temperature among varying urine flow rates. The study took place in a tertiary care center in western Washington state and included a convenience sample of 60 patients receiving cardiac surgery. This pretest-posttest quasi-experimental design included data collection over five months from 60 subjects in 2 groups: 35 from an intervention group and 25 from a control group. The intervention consisted of an intravenous diuretic, furosemide [Lasix], administered once postoperatively. The researcher measured urinary bladder temperature (UBT), pulmonary artery temperature (PAT), and urine flow rates every 2 minutes for 60 minutes both pre and post diuretic administration. Fallis (2005) concluded that bladder temperature is an applicable measurement of temperature in the critical care unit, as it is reflective of body temperature.

Relevant Study Results

In Table I, Fallis (2005) presents the socio-demographic characteristics of the sample by group: the intervention or treatment group and the control group. In Table II, the urinary bladder temperature (UBT), pulmonary artery temperature (PAT), and the difference between the two temperatures for both the intervention and control group are presented. Reported results include a significant increase in urine flow rate and a significant decrease in the UBT-PAT gradient. The researcher states that these results are significant but not "clinically important," indicating "that bladder temperature remains reliable even with significant changes in urine flow rate" (Fallis, 2005, p. 209).

TABLE I ■ Comparison of Intervention and Control Groups (*N* = 60)*			
Variable	Intervention group (*n* = 35)	Control group (*n* = 25)	*p*
Age (y)	64.34 (13.24)	62.64 (17.67)	0.671
Height (cm)	175.11 (6.80)	172.24 (9.81)	0.185
Weight (kg)	88.08 (15.54)	80.32 (20.83)	0.103
BSA (m²)	2.03 (0.18)	1.93 (0.26)	0.081
BMI (kg/m²)	28.77 (5.10)	27.02 (6.73)	0.258
SEX			0.556
Male	27 (77)	17 (68)	
Female	8 (23)	8 (32)	
SURGICAL PROCEDURE			0.378
CABG	24 (69)	11 (44)	
Aortic valve replacement/repair	4 (11)	4 (16)	
Mitral valve replacement/repair	2 (6)	2 (8)	
CABG + valve replacement/repair	1 (3)	3 (12)	
Other	4 (11)	5 (20)	

BSA, body surface area; *BMI*, body mass index; *CABG*, coronary artery bypass graft.
*All values are means (standard deviation) except sex and surgical procedure, which are reported as frequency (%).
Fallis, W. M. (2005). The effect of urine flow rate on urinary bladder temperature in critically ill adults. *Heart & Lung, 34*(3), p. 212.

TABLE II ■ Urinary Bladder Temperature, Pulmonary Artery Temperature, and Urinary Bladder Minus Pulmonary Artery Temperature Gradient for Intervention and Control Groups (N = 60)

	INTERVENTION GROUP (n = 35)			CONTROL GROUP (n = 25)		
Phase	UBT (°C)	PAT (°C)	UBT – PAT Gradient (°C)	UBT (°C)	PAT (°C)	UBT – PAT Gradient (°C)
PREPHASE						
Mean (SD)	37.49 (0.41)	37.17 (0.40)	0.32 (0.14)	37.63 (0.38)	37.28 (0.36)	0.35 (0.15)
Range	36.51 – 38.35	36.17 – 38.12	0.07 – 0.62	36.61 – 38.63	36.48 – 38.22	0.04 – 0.61
POSTPHASE						
Mean (SD)	37.34 (3.39)	37.11 (0.37)	0.23 (0.12)	37.53 (0.37)	37.18 (0.35)	0.35 (0.24)
Range	36.11 – 38.21	36.21 – 38.08	0.02 – 0.54	36.81 – 38.54	36.17 – 38.24	0.03 – 0.56
POSTPHASE MINUS Prophase						
Mean (SD)	−0.15 (0.16)	−0.06 (0.12)	−0.09 (SEM = 0.02)*	−0.10 (0.16)	−0.10 (0.14)	0.00 (SEM = 0.02)†
95 % CI			−0.13 – 0.06			−0.04 – 0.03

CI, Confidence interval; *UBT*, urinary bladder temperature; *PAT*, pulmonary artery temperature; *SD*, standard deviation; *SEM*, standard error of mean.
*$p < 0.001$, prephase compared with postphase.
†$p = 0.001$, intervention compared with control group.
Fallis, W. M. (2005). The effect of urine flow rate on urinary bladder temperature in critically ill adults. *Heart & Lung, 34*(3), p. 213.

■ STUDY QUESTIONS

1. List the different types of analysis techniques commonly used to describe variables that are measured at the interval/ratio level.

2. Identify the variables in Table I that are measured at the interval/ratio level. Can you determine if the variables are measured at the interval or ratio level? Provide a rationale for your answer.

3. Examine Table I. What descriptive analysis techniques are used to describe the variables measured at the interval/ratio level?

4. Describe interval and ratio levels of measurement.

5. Give an example of a variable measured at the interval level. Provide a rationale for your answer.

6. Give an example of a variable measured at the ratio level. Provide a rationale for your answer.

7. At what level of measurement is the variable sex or gender? Provide a rationale for your answer.

8. Discuss the purposes of parametric analyses.

9. The researcher reports "no significant differences were noted between the sample ($N = 60$) and the population of patients undergoing cardiac surgery over a similar time frame during the previous year ($N = 395$)" (Fallis, 2005, p. 211). What do "significant results" mean in a study? Should the results of this study be generalized? Provide a rationale for your answer.

■ ANSWERS TO STUDY QUESTIONS

1. Analysis techniques commonly used to describe variables measured at the interval/ratio level include: means, standard deviations, and range. Mode, frequency, and percentage (%) are used to describe variables measured at the nominal level; median, range, and often frequencies and percentages are used to describe variables measured at the ordinal level.

2. The variables age, height, weight, BSA (body surface area), and BMI (body mass index) meet the criteria for interval/ratio level of measurement. Actually these variables are measured at the ratio level since the distances between the intervals on the scales are numerically equal and the variables have an absolute zero.

3. Descriptive analysis techniques used to analyze the variables measured at the interval/ratio level in Table I are means and standard deviations.

4. With interval level measurement, the distances between the intervals of the scale are numerically equal; however, the variable with interval level of measurement has no absolute zero (0) point where the property does not exist. Ratio level measurement meets the criteria for interval level of measurement and also has an absolute zero (0) where the property does not exist.

5. Examples of variables measured at the interval level include temperature measurements of Celsius and Fahrenheit. Zero (0) degree Centigrade or 0 degree Fahrenheit indicate that the temperature is very cold but the temperature exists at 0. So temperature does not have an absolute zero (0) where there is an absence of temperature.

6. Variables measured at the ratio level have continuous values with equal distance spaces between each of the values and an absolute zero point where the property does not exist. Examples of variables measured at the ratio level include: weight, height, respirations, pulse, blood pressure, fasting blood sugar, and total cholesterol, where 0 weight means no weight or the absence of weight and 0 blood pressure means no blood pressure.

7. Sex or gender is a variable that is measured at the nominal level. The variable sex has two distinct categories (male and female) that are exhaustive for gender and mutually exclusive; the subjects can only fit into one category but the categories cannot be rank ordered.

8. Parametric statistical analysis techniques are usually used to analyze interval and ratio level data to describe study variables, examine relationships among variables, and determine differences between groups.

9. Answers may vary. Significant results are those in keeping with the outcomes predicted by the researcher, where the null hypothesis is rejected. Significant results are usually identified by * or p values $\leq$ alpha (α), which is often set at 0.05 for a study. So any p values ≤ 0.05 are considered significant. With the information provided, these research findings might be generalized to the population of patients undergoing cardiac surgery. However, it would be unwise to generalize the results of this study to other populations, meaning those that differed in age, gender, disease conditions, or surgeries, from this population.

■ EXERCISE 3   Questions to be Graded

1. List the levels of measurement from lowest to highest.

2. Identify an analysis technique that is used to examine relationships between variables measured at the interval/ratio level.

3. Which variables in Table II are measured at the interval/ratio level? Provide a rationale for your answer.

4. Which level of measurement, interval or ratio, has an absolute zero point? What does an absolute zero point mean?

5. What is the level of measurement of the three variables in Table II? Do these variables have an absolute zero point? Provide a rationale for your answer.

6. Looking at Table II, what descriptive analysis techniques were performed on the interval/ratio data?

7. In Table I, what level of measurement is the variable surgical procedure? Provide a rationale for your answer.

8. Examine Table II and list the parametric statistical analysis techniques that are included. What is a parametric analysis technique, and when is it used?

9. Are there significant differences between the intervention and the control groups for any of the variables in Table I? Provide a rationale for your answer.

10. You could measure pulse rate as slow (less than 65), moderate (65–90), or fast (greater than 90). Or, you could actually report the specific pulse rate for each subject after taking his or her pulse for a minute and the pulses might be 76 for one subject, 68 for another, and 82 for another. What was the level of measurement for pulse as slow, moderate, and fast? What is the level of measurement for a specific pulse for each subject? Which level of measurement would be the strongest to use in a study? Provide a rationale for your answer.

UNDERSTANDING PERCENTAGES

STATISTICAL TECHNIQUE IN REVIEW

Percentage can be defined as a portion of the whole, or a named amount in every hundred parts. The percentage is calculated by dividing the smaller number, which would be a part of the whole, by the larger number, which represents the whole. The result of this calculation is then multiplied by 100%. For example, if 14 nurses out of a total of 62 are working on a given day, you can divide 14 by 62 and multiply by 100% to calculate the percentage of nurses working on that day. Calculations: $14 \div 62 = 0.2258 \times 100\% = 22.58\% = 22.6\%$ or 23%.

RESEARCH ARTICLE

Source: Brawarsky, P., Brooks, D. R., & Mucci, L. A. (2003). Correlates of colorectal cancer testing in Massachusetts's men and women. *Preventive Medicine, 36*(2006), pp. 659–68.

Introduction

In order to evaluate the correlation of current colorectal cancer (CRC) testing among individuals age 50 and older, researchers used questionnaire data from the 1999 Massachusetts Behavioral Risk Factor Surveillance System (MA BRFSS) and a call-back survey on colorectal cancer screening. The study explored the "gender differences in CRC testing, within a range of personal characteristics, health care characteristics, and beliefs" (Brawarsky et al., 2003, p. 660).

Relevant Study Results

A total of 1,657 of the MA BRFSS respondents were willing to be recontacted for this study. Of those, 48 were excluded because of delays in completion of their BRFSS interview. Of the remaining 1,609 individuals, 891 were reached and agreed to participate in the CRC survey, 251 refused to be interviewed, and another 239 could not be reached by phone. Another 14% could not be reached because of changes in living situations and telephone numbers. Twenty-two individuals had to be excluded from the study because they had been diagnosed with another cancer and did not want to participate. The final sample size was 869.

The researchers found that 61% of the overall survey population had a current CRC test, which was higher than the rates of CRC screening in other studies. They also found that when health care providers recommended to both men and women that they participate in the CRC testing, there was a higher incidence of testing. Men were more likely to be recommended for testing by health care providers and were more likely to receive CRC testing. Men were more likely to have a colonoscopy or sigmoidoscopy than women when the procedures were recommended by their health care providers. The prevalence of CRC screening among adults age 50 and older, both overall and by type of test using the CRC call-back survey in 1999, is represented in Table 2 (Brawarsky, Brooks, & Mucci, 2003).

TABLE 2 ■ Prevalence of CRC Testing Among Adults Age 50 and Older, Overall and by Type of Test, CRC Call-Back Survey, 1999

	ALL SUBJECTS		MEN		WOMEN	
	N	% test	N	% test	N	% test
PREVALENCE						
Current test	521	60.7	214	65.6	307	57.6
Tested, not current	134	15.6	37	11.3	97	18.2
Never tested	204	23.7	75	23.0	129	24.2
TEST TYPE						
*FOBT only	121		37	17.3	84	27.4
Sigmoidoscopy/colonoscopy	353		160	74.8	193	62.9
With FOBT	154		72	45.0	82	47.7
Barium enema	47		17	7.9	30	9.8

Note: Numbers do not total 869 because of missing data.
*FOBT is annual fecal occult blood test.
Table content adapted from: Brawarsky, P., Brooks, D. R., & Mucci, L. A. (2003). Correlates of colorectal cancer testing in Massachusetts's men and women. *Preventive Medicine, 36* (2006), p. 663.

■ STUDY QUESTIONS

1. What percentage of males had a current CRC test?

2. Were males or females more up to date or current on their CRC testing?

3. What type of CRC test was performed most frequently in this sample to detect CRC? Is this what you might expect? Provide a rationale for your answer.

4. What frequency and percentage (%) of the total number of subjects had never been tested for CRC? Do you find this result to be unusual? Provide a rationale for your answer.

5. Of the procedures conducted for CRC screening, what percentage (%) was for the FOBT (fecal occult blood test) only?

6. What was the difference, as a percentage (%), between total respondents never tested for CRC and those with a current CRC test?

7. In the CRC test types for both men and women, do the percentages (%) add up to more than 100%? If so, explain why.

8. Which CRC testing type was used the least frequently by women?

9. 251 of the 1,609 eligible respondents were reached but were not willing to be interviewed. What percentage (%) of the eligible respondents did this represent? Round to the nearest % point.

10. Colorectal cancer is one of the leading causes of cancer-related death in the United States. Why is this type of cancer so prevalent in this country?

■ ANSWERS TO STUDY QUESTIONS

1. The percentage of males who had a current CRC test was 65.6%. This information is found in Table 2.

2. Males were more up to date on their CRC testing. The percentage of males with current CRC testing was 65.6% and the percentage of females was 57.6%.

3. Sigmoidoscopy/colonoscopy was performed most frequently since 353 of these procedures were conducted (see Table 2). Yes, you might expect the sigmoidoscopy/colonoscopy to be the most common procedure performed since the evidence-based national practice recommendation is for all persons over age 50 to be tested for CRC with a colonoscopy or sigmoidoscopy (http://www.ahcpr.gov). Colonoscopy is now more commonly encouraged for CRC screening than a sigmoidoscopy. However, one would expect the test for FOBT to occur with each annual physical for men and women, which would mean that the number of these procedures could have been much higher than the $N = 121$ listed for this study. In fact, FOBT might have been the most common CRC screening procedure conducted.

4. 204 subjects or 23.7% of the sample had never been tested for CRC. This is not unusual since many people (men and women) are not receiving annual physicals or participating in preventive screening for CRC. The reasons for not receiving CRC screening might be: lack of insurance and the costs of screening procedures; fear of the procedures; fear of something being found; lack of time; and health not being a high priority.

5. 121 FOBT-only procedures were performed, which was 17.93% of the procedures conducted for CRC testing. Calculations: 121 FOBT ÷ 675 total CRC procedures (121 + 353 + 154 + 47) = 0.1793 x 100% = 17.93% or 17.9% or 18%.

6. The difference, as a percentage of the total, between the total respondents never tested and those with a current test was 37%. Subtract the 23.7% of never tested from the 60.7% current CRC testing. Calculation: 60.7% − 23.7% = 37%.

7. Men % of tests was 145% (17.3% + 74.8% + 45% + 7.9%). Women % of tests was 147.8% (27.4% + 62.9% + 47.7% + 9.8%). When examining the CRC test types, the total adds up to more than 100% because some people had more than one test done. The FOBT test can be used as an initial screening test, and if positive, a sigmoidoscopy/colonoscopy is used for further screening. FOBT also could have been done prior to barium enema.

8. The least frequently used CRC testing procedure for women was barium enema with a frequency of 30 and 9.8%.

9. The answer is 16%. The number of eligible respondents was 1609 (1657 − 48). Calculations: 251 ÷ 1609 = 0.156 × 100% = 15.6 % = 16%.

10. Possible reasons for the prevalence of CRC in the United States and other developed countries include: a diet that is high in refined foods and fats and low in fiber; smoking; and a sedentary lifestyle. In addition, family history can be used as an indicator for those at high risk for CRC. Since 23.7% of the subjects in this study have never had CRC testing, this can result in late detection of CRC and increased morbidity and mortality related to this disease.

■ EXERCISE 4   Questions to be Graded

1. What number and percentage of females had never been tested for CRC?

2. Which gender group is more likely, according to this study, to have never received any CRC testing?

3. Which test was performed least often to detect CRC for the total sample, and what was its percentage (%) of the total CRC testing procedures performed?

4. What number and percentage (%) of the total number of respondents had a current CRC test?

5. What percentage (%) of the total CRC testing procedures was sigmoidoscopy/colonoscopy?

6. Explain why the number of total subjects' data in Table 2 is for 859 subjects when the total sample for the study was 869 subjects.

7. What number and percentage (%) of the qualified MA BRFSS respondents were excluded because of delays in completion of the interview? Round to the nearest % point.

8. What number and percentage (%) of the 1,609 potential subjects could not be reached by phone? Round to the nearest % point.

9. In general terms, what do the results of this study tell us about prevalence in CRC screening in this sample?

10. This study found that men are more likely to be advised by their health care provider to obtain screening for CRC. Why do you think this is happening, and how does it affect the CRC outcomes for men and women?

FREQUENCY DISTRIBUTIONS WITH PERCENTAGES

STATISTICAL TECHNIQUE IN REVIEW

Frequency distributions are used to organize the data prior to detailed examination and can be used to determine errors in coding or computer programming (Burns & Grove, 2005). Percentage distributions give an overview of the data and indicate where the subjects' scores are located. In data analysis, percentage distributions can be used to compare findings from different studies that have different sample sizes. The percentage distributions are usually arranged in tables in order either from greatest to least or least to greatest percentages.

RESEARCH ARTICLE

Source: Patistea, E., & Babatsikou, F. (2003). Parents' perceptions of the information provided to them about their child's leukemia. *European Journal of Oncology Nursing, 7*(3), 172-81.

Introduction

Patistea and Babatsikou (2003) conducted a study that included both quantitative (descriptive correlational design) and qualitative methods. They examined the type of information that was provided to parents of children in Greece who were diagnosed with leukemia. They also determined where the parents received their information, their level of satisfaction with the information received, and what additional information the parents wanted to receive.

Relevant Study Results

The subjects of the study consisted of 41 mothers, 30 fathers, and 42 children. Of the parents, 29 were couples, 12 were single mothers, and 1 was a single father. The researchers interviewed the parents either in the oncology clinic (91.5%) or in the parent's home (8.5%). The subjects were given two questionnaires, which were constructed and tested prior to the study. The results showed that the parents received information mostly about the biomedical aspects of their child's leukemia, that the majority relied on the medical staff for their information, that about half of the parents were satisfied with the information that they received, and that they wanted information on the psychosocial aspects of the disease.

The researchers found that there was little difference in the amount of information received between genders, and that those who lived in large cites with over 1,000,000 people received more information than those who lived in smaller cities or villages. They found that persons of higher educational level reported being less satisfied with the amount of information that they received, but that those who had previous experience with cancer were more satisfied with the information that they were given. There was no significant relationship between the perceived amount of information received and the seriousness of the child's illness.

Areas that were identified by the parents where more information would have been helpful included: causes of the child's illness, telling and disciplining healthy siblings, operational routine of the health care system, discipline of the child with leukemia, management of their own emotional reaction, and family planning. Table 1 shows the frequency distributions of certain characteristics of the subjects and their children, and Table 4 shows the frequency distributions of the levels of satisfaction with the information received (Patistea & Babatsikou, 2003).

TABLE 1 ■ Demographic Data of the Parents (N=71) and the Children with Leukemia (N=42)

	MOTHERS		FATHERS	
	n	%	n	%
CHARACTERISTICS OF THE PARENTS				
Level of education				
Elementary school	12	29.2	10	33.3
High school	20	48.8	10	33.3
College	4	9.8	3	10.0
University/postgraduate studies	5	12.2	7	23.4
Professional status				
Self-employed	4	9.8	13	43.3
Clerks	9	22.0	16	53.3
Housewives	28	68.3	–	–
Retired	–	–	1	3.4
Place of living				
<10,000	17	41.5	12	40.0
10,000–1,000,000	19	46.3	13	43.3
>1,000,000	5	12.2	5	16.7

	n	%
CHARACTERISTICS OF THE CHILDREN WITH LEUKEMIA		
Sex		
Boys	18	42.8
Girls	24	57.2
Type of leukemia		
Acute lymphocytic	37	88.0
Acute myelocytic	5	12.0
Stage of disease		
Continuous remission	30	71.4
Relapse	12	28.6

Patistea, E., & Babatsikou, F. (2003). Parents' perceptions of the information provided to them about their child's leukemia. *European Journal of Oncology Nursing, 7*(3), p. 176.

TABLE 4 ■ Sample's Frequency Distributions and Percentages by Level of Satisfaction (N=71)

	MOTHERS		FATHERS		SAMPLE	
	n	%	n	%	n	%
LEVEL OF SATISFACTION						
Very satisfied	7	17.1	5	16.7	12	16.9
Satisfied	15	36.6	10	33.3	25	35.2
Slightly satisfied	13	31.7	8	26.7	21	29.6
Not satisfied	6	14.6	7	23.3	13	18.3

Patistea, E., & Babatsikou, F. (2003). Parents' perceptions of the information provided to them about their child's leukemia. *European Journal of Oncology Nursing, 7*(3), p. 177.

■ STUDY QUESTIONS

1. How many mothers were self-employed, and what percentage is this of the professional status variable?

2. What frequency and percentage of the fathers live in an area of <10,000 people?

3. How many of the total subjects, the mothers, and the fathers were not satisfied with the information that they received? Give your answer as both a frequency and percent.

4. List other types of demographic variables that would have been appropriate for the researchers to gather data on to describe this sample.

5. The researchers found that the primary source of information was the physician and that the information was of a biomedical nature. What other information might be provided by nurses and other health care professionals to assist families with children with leukemia?

6. In Table 4, all of the percentage columns add up to what total percentage? What does this mean?

7. This study was a retrospective study, which means that the questionnaires were given to the subjects after they had received the information. What are some limitations to the collection of data for retrospective studies?

8. The researchers found that the parents with higher levels of education were less satisfied with the information received. Give possible reasons for this.

9. The article states that the higher the parents' educational level, the less satisfied they were with the information received. Using Tables 1 and 4, can we determine the educational level of all the persons not satisfied with the information received?

◼ ANSWERS TO STUDY QUESTIONS

1. The answer is 4 mothers, which is 9.8% of the professional status variable. The information on mothers who are self-employed is found in Table 1.
2. The answer is 12 fathers, which is 40% of the variable place of living. The frequency and percent of fathers who live in an area of <10,000 people is found in Table 1.
3. Table 4 identifies the level of satisfaction for mothers, fathers, and the total sample. In this study, 6 (14.6%) of the mothers, 7 (23.3%) of the fathers, and 13 (18.3%) of the total sample were not satisfied with the information they received.
4. Possible answers include: ethnicity of parents and children, age of parents and children, socioeconomic status, number of siblings, and other medical diagnoses.
5. Nurses, physicians, and other health care professionals need to be knowledgeable of and provide more information to parents and children on: the emotional aspects of major illnesses, the disease process, the psychosocial and spiritual aspects of health and illness, ways to cope with illness, and costs related to care. It is best for an interdisciplinary team to work with parents in caring for their seriously ill children.
6. In a percentage distribution, all of the data must fit into a category, and no data should be placed in more than one category. Thus, if no data are missing, the categories should add up to 100%. All three percentages columns (mothers, fathers, and sample) add up to 100%.
7. Recall of information produces less accurate and complete data than gathering data during or immediately after an event. The subjects may have forgotten some of their first reactions to a situation or event. There has also been time for the subjects to forget information that they may have received when their children were first diagnosed. This often happens when a great deal of information is given at a time of increased stress.
8. Pathophysiology and biomedical aspects of care are discussed to the extent that it is known, but much is still unknown about leukemia. Many aspects of the disease are not discussed, such as the psychological, social, and spiritual dimensions, because the health care providers lack the knowledge and the comfort level to provide this type of information. This increases the frustration and stress in a population which is used to gaining insights through education.
9. No, not by looking at the two tables. The 13 people in Table 4 who were not satisfied are part of the total sample but are not clearly linked to a particular educational group. The only way to link educational level to satisfaction level is through examining the raw data for each subject.

■ EXERCISE 5   Questions to be Graded

1. What number and percentage of the children were diagnosed with acute lymphocytic leukemia?

2. Identify the frequency and percentage of fathers who had attained either a high school education or higher.

3. How many more mothers (frequency and percentage) were housewives than were clerks?

4. What level of education achieved by the mothers is the mode for this variable? Document your answer as both a frequency and percentage.

5. Were the mothers or fathers more "Satisfied" with the information that they received? Express your answer as both a frequency and a percentage.

6. Only 3.4% of the fathers were retired. Is this an unlikely finding? Provide a rationale for your answer.

7. Using the rule for frequency distribution, if 20 children were in continuous remission, how many and what percentage would be in relapse based on the sample size of this study?

8. The article states that $^1/_5$ or 20% of the parents had a previous experience with cancer information. How could this affect the results of the study?

9. The study indicated that parents in larger cities received more information as compared to those living in smaller cities, towns, or villages. Give possible reasons for this.

10. Do you think that this study and its results can be generalized to the United States? Provide a rationale for your answer.

6

CUMULATIVE PERCENTAGES AND PERCENTILE RANKS

STATISTICAL TECHNIQUE IN REVIEW

A **cumulative percentage distribution** involves the summing of percentages from the top of a table to the bottom. Therefore, the bottom category has a cumulative percentage of 100. Cumulative percentages can also be used to determine percentile ranks, especially when discussing standardized test scores. For example, if 75% of a group scored equal to or lower than a particular examinee's score, then that examinee's rank is at the 75th percentile. When reported as a percentile rank, the percentage is often rounded to a whole number. Percentile ranks can be used to analyze ordinal data that can be assigned to categories able to be ranked. Percentile ranks and cumulative percentages are often applied to exam scores, but may be used in any frequency distribution where subjects have only one value for a variable. For example, demographic characteristics are usually reported with the frequency (f) or number (n) of subjects and percentage of subjects (%) for each level of a demographic variable. Income level for 200 subjects is presented as an example.

Income Level	Frequency (f)	Percentage (%)	Cumulative %
1. < $40,000	20	10	10
2. $40,000–59,999	50	25	35
3. $60,000–79,999	80	40	75
4. $80,000–100,000	40	20	95
5. > $100,000	10	5	100

RESEARCH ARTICLE

Source: Katsma, D. L., & Souza, C. H. (2000). Elderly pain assessment and pain management knowledge of long-term care nurses. *Pain Management Nursing, 1*(3), 88–95.

Introduction

Katsma and Souza (2000) conducted a descriptive study using a convenience sample of long-term care nurses from six rural counties in California to evaluate the nurses' knowledge base of assessment and management of pain in the elderly. Questionnaires were mailed to selected nursing homes and 89 nurses responded. The nurses reviewed two scenarios and responded to questions related to these scenarios. The scenarios were identical, except one involved a smiling patient and the other a grimacing patient. The researchers found that the nurses surveyed "were more likely to believe and document the grimacing patient's self-report of pain than the smiling patient" (Katsma & Souza, 2003, p. 88). Fewer than half of the respondents chose to increase the analgesic dose for either patient scenario. "Nursing implications include the importance of ongoing pain assessment and management education tailored to the geriatric population and in long term care" (Katsma & Souza, 2000, p. 88).

Relevant Study Results

Three tables adapted from Katsma and Souza's (2000) study are presented in this section. The tables address the research questions and include the number (*n*) and percent (%) of the nurses' assessment of elders' pain score and their medication management of that pain. The tables might have been clearer if an *f* had been used for frequencies versus the *n*. Tables 1a and 1b contain the nurses' private opinions and documentations of their assessment of the patients' self-reported pain score. Table 2 shows the numbers and percentages of nurses' medication choices for the management of the elders' pain score. The younger nurses with less clinical experience were more likely to believe and document their patients' self-report of pain and to manage that pain with medication than the older more experienced nurses (Katsma & Souza, 2000).

TABLE 1a ■ Nurses' Belief and Documentation of Assessment of the Smiling Patient

Pain Assessment Scale	OPINION			DOCUMENTATION		
	n	%	Cumulative %	*N*	%	Cumulative %
0	7	8.1	8.1	3	3.5	3.5
1	7	8.1	16.2	5	5.8	9.3
2	5	5.8	22.0	6	7.0	16.3
3	8	9.4	31.4	4	4.7	21.0
4	10	11.6	43.0	4	4.7	25.7
5	11	12.8	55.8	7	8.0	33.7
6	5	5.8	61.6	1	1.2	34.9
7	2	2.3	63.9	0	0.0	34.9
8*	31	36.1	100.0	56	65.1	100.0
9	0	0.0	100.0	0	0.0	100.0
10	0	0.0	100.0	0	0.0	100.0

* Correct Answer.
Adapted from Katsma, D. L., & Souza, C. H. (2000). Elderly pain assessment and pain management knowledge of long-term care nurses. *Pain Management Nursing, 1*(3), p. 91. Copyright © 2000 with permission from The American Society for Pain Management Nursing.

TABLE 1b ■ Nurses' Belief and Documentation of Assessment of the Grimacing Patient

Pain Assessment Scale	OPINION			DOCUMENTATION		
	n	%	Cumulative %	*N*	%	Cumulative %
0	0	0.0	0.0	0	0.0	0.0
1	0	0.0	0.0	0	0.0	0.0
2	1	1.2	1.2	1	1.2	1.2
3	1	1.2	2.4	1	1.2	2.4
4	1	1.2	3.6	1	1.2	3.6
5	4	4.7	8.3	4	4.7	8.3
6	8	9.3	17.6	7	8.0	16.3
7	8	9.3	26.9	3	3.5	19.8
8*	48	55.8	82.7	60	69.8	89.6
9	8	9.3	92.0	6	7.0	96.6
10	7	8.0	100.0	3	3.4	100.0

* Correct Answer.
Adapted from Katsma, D. L., & Souza, C. H. (2000). Elderly pain assessment and pain management knowledge of long-term care nurses. *Pain Management Nursing, 1*(3), p. 91. Copyright © 2000 with permission from The American Society for Pain Management Nursing.

TABLE 2 ■ Nurses' Medication Choice

Medication Choice	SMILING PATIENT			GRIMACING PATIENT		
	n	%	Cumulative %	n	%	Cumulative %
No pain medication now	9	10.5	10.5	0	0.0	0.0
Extra Strength Tylenol	17	19.8	30.3	2	2.3	2.3
Vicodin 1 Tablet	33	38.4	68.7	37	43.0	45.3
Vicodin 2 Tablets*	26	30.1	98.8	47	54.7	100.0
Response Missing	1	1.2	100.0	0	0.0	100.0

* Correct Answer.
Adapted from Katsma, D. L., & Souza, C. H. (2000). Elderly pain assessment and pain management knowledge of long-term care nurses. *Pain Management Nursing, 1*(3), p. 92. Copyright © 2000 with permission from The American Society for Pain Management Nursing.

■ STUDY QUESTIONS

1. What number and percentage of nurses documented the correct pain assessment score for the grimacing patient?

2. What number of nurses and cumulative percentage of nurses had an opinion lower than the self-reported pain score of the smiling patient?

3. How many nurses undermedicated the smiling patient?

4. What cumulative percentage of nurses undermedicated the grimacing patient?

5. What number of nurses and percentage of nurses chose the correct medication plan for the grimacing patient?

6. How many nurses had an opinion that differed from the grimacing patient's self-report of a pain score of 8?

7. What cumulative percentage of nurses' opinions was that the grimacing patient was in less pain than reported?

8. What number and percentage of nurses documented the smiling patient's pain score at or below 6?

9. What percentage of nurses documented a pain score higher than the correct score for the grimacing patient? Compare that percentage with the percentage of nurses whose opinion was that the grimacing patient was in more pain than reported.

10. Why do you think so many nurses undermedicated the grimacing patient?

▨ ANSWERS TO STUDY QUESTIONS

1. 60 nurses or 69.8% of the nurses documented a pain score of 8 for the grimacing patient. The key for Table 1b indicates that * designates the correct answer; thus 8* is the correct pain score for the grimacing patient.

2. 55 nurses or 63.9% of the nurses had the opinion that the smiling patient's actual pain was less than his self-report. The 63.9% is obtained from Table 1a, and the figure of 55 nurses is obtained by adding the number of nurses whose opinions were that the pain score was less than 8 or those who gave a score of 0 to 7.

3. 59 nurses undermedicated the smiling patient. This number is obtained by adding the number of nurses giving no pain medication (9), the number giving extra-strength Tylenol (17), and the number giving 1 tablet of Vicodin (33), which equals 59 nurses.

4. 45.3% of nurses undermedicated the grimacing patient, which is found in Table 2.

5. 47 nurses or 54.7% chose to medicate the grimacing patient with 2 Vicodin tablets, which was the correct choice of medication indicated in Table 2.

6. 38 nurses' opinions differed from the self-report of an 8 pain score by the grimacing patient. This number is found by adding the number of nurses who had an opinion that the pain score was less than 8, which was 23 nurses, and those nurses who thought the pain score was greater than 8, which was 15 nurses. Thus, 23 + 15 = 38 nurses' opinions differed from the reported pain score of 8 (see Table 1b).

7. 26.9% of nurses were of the opinion that the grimacing patient's actual pain was less than 8 (see Table 1b).

8. 30 (34.9%) of the nurses documented a pain score of 6 or less for the smiling patient (see Table 1a).

9. 10.4% of nurses documented a higher pain score than the correct score of 8. This number is obtained by adding the percent of nurses giving a score of 9 and 10. 17.3% of the nurses were of the opinion that the grimacing patient's actual pain was higher than his self-reported pain score of 8. Thus, not all the nurses who had the opinion that the patients were in more pain (17.3%) than reported documented (10.4%) his or her opinion. The difference was 17.3% – 10.4% = 6.9%.

10. Answers may vary. The grimacing patient may have been undermedicated for any of the following reasons: limited pain assessment skills of the nurse; underestimating the medication needed to treat the pain; lack of knowledge or experience with pain medications; reluctance to give narcotics to the elderly; or nurses are often very cautious about overmedicating patients, sometimes resulting in undermedication.

■ EXERCISE 6   Questions to be Graded

1. What number and percentage of nurses documented the correct pain assessment for the smiling patient?

2. What number and cumulative percentage of nurses had an opinion that the smiling patient had a 5 or lower pain score?

3. What number and percentage of nurses chose the correct medication plan for the smiling patient?

4. What number and percentage of nurses documented the pain score higher than the correct score for the smiling patient?

5. What number and percentage of nurses documented a different pain score from the grimacing patient's self-reported pain score of 8?

6. What cumulative percentage of nurses' opinions was that the smiling patient was in less pain than reported?

7. What number and percentage of the nurses documented the grimacing patient's pain score at or below 6?

8. Why do you think so many nurses undermedicated the smiling patient?

9. Is this study only applicable to the elderly population? Do you think younger patients' self-reports of pain are believed and their pain appropriately treated?

10. What can you learn from this study for your practice?

INTERPRETING HISTOGRAMS

STATISTICAL TECHNIQUE IN REVIEW

Figures provide the reader with a picture of the results of a study and are used to support the major points of a research project. Common figures include bar and line graphs. Bar graphs have horizontal or vertical bars, and a **histogram** is a bar graph consisting of vertical bars. Continuous variables are placed on the horizontal or *x*-axis, and the vertical or *y*-axis measures the occurrence with frequencies or percentages. The mode, a descriptive statistic, is visible on the histogram, since it is the most frequently occurring score. Also visible on a histogram is the distribution pattern, and a normal distribution pattern follows a bell-shaped curve. Data that occur outside of the distribution pattern are considered outliers (Burns & Grove, 2005).

A **normal or bell-shaped curve** is symmetrical, meaning the left side of the curve mirrors the right side. A curve that is not symmetrical means that the left side does not mirror the right side. A non-normal curve is referred to as asymmetrical or skewed. Skewness is a shift in the distribution that leads to outliers and often interferes with statistical analysis (Burns & Grove, 2005). Please refer to Exercise 19 for additional information regarding skewness.

RESEARCH ARTICLE

Source: Schaffner, B., & Vogt, M. (2004). Pediatric nurse practitioner practice patterns and compensation in Ohio. *Journal of Pediatric Health Care, 18*(4), 180–5.

Introduction

In an effort to "describe practice and compensation patterns of Pediatric Nurse Practitioners (PNPs) in Ohio," Schaffner and Vogt (2004) surveyed all members of Ohio's chapter of the National Association of Pediatric Nurse Practitioners and Associates (NAPNAP) (Schaffner & Vogt, 2004, p. 180). The study included 156 female PNPs with 1–36 years of practice experience. Important sample characteristics include a PNP average age of 45–55, and 59.8% reporting full-time work status. A total of 18% of the participating PNPs took on-call time, approximately 38% were practicing in a private practice, and 38% were practicing in a hospital setting. Findings include a gross annual salary ranging from $35,000 to $90,000 per year and hourly wages ranging from $19.00 to $40.00 per hour. It is important to note that the authors report that the practice patterns of Ohio's PNPs were similar to the practice patterns of other advanced practice nurses across the United States.

Relevant Study Results

Of the sample population, 59.8% reported working full-time, 38.5% reported working part-time, and 1.5% reported working on an as-needed basis. Only 21.8% of the sample population reported billing under their own names. In the state of Ohio, PNPs are required to have a collaborative agreement with a physician. In Figure 1, Schaffner and Vogt (2004) presented the gross annual Ohio PNP salaries, and in Figure 2, they included the Ohio PNP hourly wages (Schaffner & Vogt, 2004).

FIGURE 1 ■ Gross annual Ohio PNP salaries ($n = 78$)

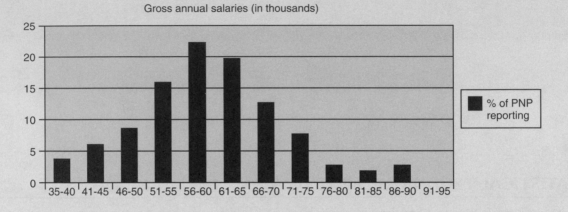

FIGURE 2 ■ Ohio PNP hourly wages ($n = 42$)

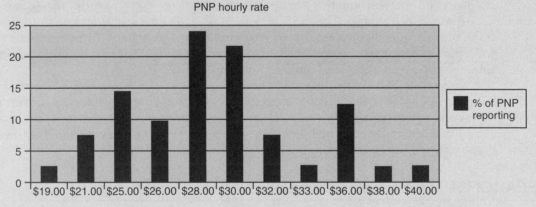

(Schaffner, B., & Vogt, M. (2004). Pediatric nurse practitioner practice patterns and compensation in Ohio. *Journal of Pediatric Health Cares, 18*(4), p. 183. Copyright © 2004 with permission from The National Association of Pediatric Nurses.)

◼ STUDY QUESTIONS

1. In Figure 1, what percentage of the Ohio Pediatric Nurse Practitioners (PNPs) reported earning a gross annual salary between $51,000 and $55,000?

2. In Figure 1, what percentage of the Ohio PNPs reported earning a gross annual salary between $41,000 and $50,000?

3. In Figure 1, which gross annual salary was reported most frequently by Ohio PNPs?

4. In Figure 1, which gross annual salary is the mode? Provide a rationale for your answer.

5. In Figure 1, which reported gross annual salary does not fit the normal distribution pattern? Provide a rationale for your answer.

6. Using the information found in Figure 1, calculate the actual number of the Ohio PNPs who earned a salary between $61,000 and $65,000.

7. What is the distribution pattern of Figure 1? Is it normal or skewed? Provide a rationale for your answer.

8. In Figure 1, which variable is placed on the x-axis and which is placed on the y-axis?

9. This study included the practice patterns of female PNPs. In your own opinion, do you think that this study should have included male PNPs as well? If male participants were included, might the compensation rates differ?

ANSWERS TO STUDY QUESTIONS

1. In Figure 1, approximately 16%, or slightly over 15%, of the Ohio PNPs reported earning a gross annual salary between $51,000 and $55,000.
2. In Figure 1, approximately 6% of Ohio PNPs reported earning a gross annual salary between $41,000 and $45,000, and 8% reported earning a gross annual salary between $46,000 and $50,000. Therefore 14% of Ohio PNPs reported earning a gross annual salary between $41,000 and $50,000.
3. In Figure 1, a gross annual salary between $56,000 and $60,000 was reported most frequently by Ohio PNPs.
4. The gross annual salary of $56,000–$60,000 is the mode or the most frequently reported salary by Ohio PNPs.
5. In Figure 1, the percent of PNPs who reported a salary of $86,000–$90,000 does not fit the shape of a normal curve. This distribution is not a perfect normal curve because more of the Ohio PNPs reported a salary of $86,000–$90,000 than $81,000–$85,000.
6. In Figure 1, approximately 20% of the participating Ohio PNPs reported earning a gross annual salary between $61,000 and $65,000. Using a sample size of 78, $n = 78$, the actual number of Ohio PNPs who received a gross annual salary between $61,000 and $65,000 is calculated as: 20% = 20 ÷ 100 = 0.20, and 0.20 × 78 = 15.6 or approximately 16 PNPs.
7. The pattern in Figure 1 is approximately a normal distribution, meaning the vertical bars fall into the shape of a normal bell-shaped curve. Another characteristic of a normal curve is that the mode is in the middle of the distribution and the two halves of the curve are symmetrical. A skewness analysis should be run to detect the effect of outliers on the distribution of the curve.
8. In Figure 1, gross annual salary in thousands is placed on the x or horizontal axis, and the percent of reporting PNPs is placed on the y or vertical axis.
9. Answers may vary. When analyzing compensation and practice patterns of PNPs, it is important to include both male and female PNPs. Since this article only reflects the compensation and practice patterns of female PNPs in Ohio, the title of the article might read "Female Pediatric Nurse Practitioner Practice Patterns and Compensation in Ohio." It would be interesting to discover if the compensation rates for male and female PNPs differed, as they do so often in other professions. This topic requires further research.

■ EXERCISE 7　Questions to be Graded

1. In Figure 2, what percentage of the participating Ohio PNPs reported earning a $25.00 hourly rate?

2. In Figure 2, what hourly wage or wages was or were reported least frequently by Ohio PNPs?

3. In Figure 2, what hourly wage was reported most frequently by Ohio PNPs?

4. In Figure 2, what percentage of the Ohio PNPs reported earning an hourly wage between $38.00 and $40.00?

5. In Figure 2, what hourly wage is the mode? Provide a rationale for your answer.

6. Using the information found in Figure 2, calculate the actual number of Ohio PNPs who earned an hourly wage of $28.00, which was about 24% of the PNPs.

7. In Figure 2, which variable is placed on the x-axis? Which variable is placed on the y-axis?

8. In your opinion, if more that 59.8% of Ohio PNPs reported working full-time, and more than 18% were required to take on-call time, what would happen to the compensation patterns if more PNPs worked full-time and with on-call compensation?

9. Examine Figures 1 and 2 and compare their distribution patterns. Are the distribution patterns similar? Provide a rationale for you answer.

10. Should the results of this study be generalized to other states? Provide a rationale for your answer.

INTERPRETING LINE GRAPHS

STATISTICAL TECHNIQUE IN REVIEW

Tables and figures are commonly used to present findings from a study or to provide a way for researchers to become familiar with research data (Burns & Grove, 2005). Using tables and figures, researchers are able to illustrate the results from descriptive data analyses, assist in identifying patterns in data, and interpret exploratory findings. A **line graph** is a figure that is developed by joining a series of points with a line to show how a variable changes over time. A line graph includes a horizontal scale or x-axis and a vertical scale or y-axis. The x-axis is used to document time, and the y-axis is used to document the number or quantity of a variable. Below is an example line graph that documents time in weeks on the x-axis and weight loss in pounds on the y-axis.

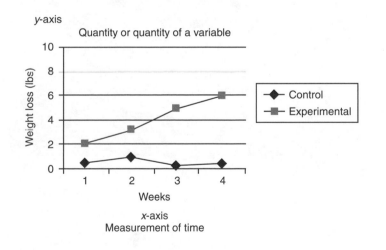

RESEARCH ARTICLE

Source: Kang, N. M., Song, Y., Hyun, T. H., & Kim, K. N. (2005). Evaluation of the breastfeeding intervention program in a Korean community health center. *International Journal of Nursing Studies, 42*(4), 409–13.

Introduction

Kang, Song, Hyun, and Kim (2005) conducted an observational study to examine a new breastfeeding intervention implemented in a Korean community health center. The purpose of the study was to determine if breastfeeding rates increased after trained health care professionals and peers gave information on breastfeeding to pregnant and lactating women. Breastfeeding rates after the educational program significantly increased, indicating that the community-based breastfeeding intervention program was effective in promoting breastfeeding among these women (Kang et al., 2005).

Relevant Study Results

The researchers presented their results in a line graph format to display outcomes comparing the pre-intervention group to the post-intervention group (see Figures 1 to 3). The x-axis represents age of the babies in months in the three figures, and the y-axis represents breastfeeding rate in Figure 1, formula-feeding rate in Figure 2, and mixed-feeding rate in Figure 3.

FIGURE 1   Breastfeeding rate of pre- and post-intervention (* Significance <0.05 by χ^2-test).

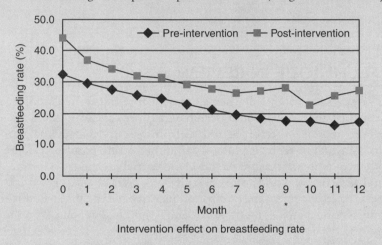

FIGURE 2   Formula-feeding rate of pre- and post-intervention (* Significance <0.05 by χ^2-test).

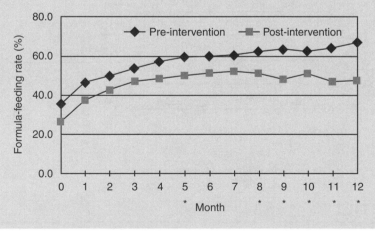

FIGURE 3 ■ Mixed-feeding rate of pre- and post-intervention.

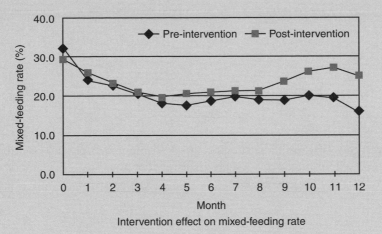

Intervention effect on mixed-feeding rate

(Figures 1 to 3 from Kang, N. M., Song, Y., Hyun, T. H., Kim, K. N. (2005), Evaluation of the breastfeeding intervention program in a Korean community health center *International Journal of Nursing Studies, 42*(4), p. 412)

■ STUDY QUESTIONS

1. Which axis shows the length of time of the study? Provide a rationale for the use of length of time in a line graph. What time interval was used in this study?

2. According to the line graphs in Figures 1–3, this study included babies up to how many months old?

3. What was the breastfeeding rate pre-intervention at 1 month?

4. What was the formula-feeding rate for babies pre-intervention at 5 months? Was this pre-intervention rate significantly different from the post-intervention rate? Provide a rationale for your answer.

5. Was there a significant difference in breastfeeding pre- and post-intervention? Provide a rationale for your answer.

6. The highest percentage of formula-feeding occurred during which pre-intervention month? Was this an expected or unexpected finding? Provide a rationale for your answer.

7. What information does Figure 1 provide you about the effectiveness of the breastfeeding educational program?

8. What percentages of 7-month-old babies were breastfed pre-intervention? Was this breastfeeding rate significantly different from the post-intervention breastfeeding rate? Provide a rationale for your answer.

9. Were formula-feeding rates affected by the intervention? Provide a rationale for your answer.

ANSWERS TO STUDY QUESTIONS

1. The x-axis of a line graph shows the length of time examined in a study. The use of time in a line graph helps you to see how a variable changes or varies over time. In this study, time was measured in months to show a trend of feeding methods used for new babies over the course of 12 months.

2. This study included babies up to 12 months old.

3. The breastfeeding rate pre-intervention was 30% for the 1-month-old infants.

4. The pre-intervention formula-feeding rate for babies at 5 months was 60%. At 5 months the pre-intervention and post-intervention rates were significantly different, as indicated by the asterisk (*) below the 5. The * indicates significant differences at $p < 0.05$.

5. Yes, at 1 month and 9 months there were significant differences in the breastfeeding rates pre- and post-intervention. This is represented by *s on the x-axis at 1 and 9 months, indicating that at these two particular months, there were significant differences in pre- and post-intervention at $p < 0.05$. The content presented from the research article indicated that breastfeeding rates after the educational program significantly increased, indicating that the community-based breastfeeding intervention program was effective in promoting breastfeeding among these women (Kang et al., 2005).

6. The highest percentage of formula-feeding occurred at 12 months pre-intervention. This is an expected finding considering that most women decrease the amount of breastfeeding to their child as the child gets older. So the 12th and final month of the study would be expected to show the highest formula-feeding rate.

7. Figure 1 indicates that breastfeeding rates for the post-intervention group were higher every month than those for the pre-intervention group. Although, no statistically significant differences were found between pre- and post-intervention breastfeeding rates, except for months 1 and 9. Thus, the findings indicate that the educational program was effective in increasing breastfeeding rates among the women, but with limited significant differences between pre- and post-intervention.

8. At 7 months pre-intervention, the breastfeeding rate was 20%, which was not significantly different from the post-intervention rate since there was no * below the month indicating a statistically significant difference. In addition, the line diagram indicates very limited difference between the pre- and post-intervention groups at 7 months.

9. Yes. When compared to pre-intervention rates, formula-feeding rates declined post-intervention at the same time that the breastfeeding rates increased. This indicates that people changed from formula-feeding to breastfeeding after the educational program.

■ EXERCISE 8   Questions to be Graded

1. Can the exact percentage for the type of feeding rate per month for the pre- and post-intervention groups be determined from the line graphs? Provide a rationale for your answer.

2. Did the breastfeeding rate decline at the 12th month post-intervention? Provide a rationale for your answer.

3. If the level of statistical significance was determined at $p < 0.05$ level for this study, at what months were the rates of formula-feeding statistically significant between pre- and post-interventions? Provide a rationale for you answer.

4. What were the trends for mixed-feeding rates post-intervention? Were these results significant? Provide a rationale for your answer.

5. At 9 months of age, the breastfeeding rate post-intervention (28%) was significantly different from the pre-intervention rate (18%). Is this statement true or false?

6. The breastfeeding rate post-intervention was greater than the pre-intervention rate over the 12 months of the study. Is this statement true or false? Provide a rationale for your answer.

7. Were the mixed-feeding rates for the pre-intervention and post-intervention groups significantly different at 7 months? Provide a rationale for your answer.

8. Do the results of this study support the hypothesis that the breastfeeding program would contribute to an increase in the breastfeeding rate in the community? Provide a rationale for you answer.

9. Were the breastfeeding rates statistically significant at 1 and 9 months of age? Provide a rationale for your answer.

10. What implications for practice do you note from these study results?

IDENTIFYING PROBABILITY AND NONPROBABILITY SAMPLING METHODS

STATISTICAL TECHNIQUE IN REVIEW

A **sampling method** is the process researchers use to select subjects from the population being studied, and sampling methods are categorized as either probability or nonprobability. Descriptions of the common probability and nonprobability sampling methods used in quantitative studies, and the nonprobability sampling methods used most frequently in qualitative studies, are discussed in this exercise.

Probability Sampling

Probability sampling, also known as random sampling, requires that every member of the study population have an equal opportunity to be chosen as a study subject. For each member of the population to have an equal opportunity to be chosen, the sampling method must select members randomly. Probability sampling allows every facet of the study population to be represented without researcher bias. Four common sampling designs have been developed for selection of a random sample: simple random sampling, stratified random sampling, cluster sampling, and systematic sampling (Burns & Grove, 2007). **Simple random sampling** is achieved by random selection of members from the sampling frame. The random selection can be accomplished many different ways, but the most common is using a computer program to randomly select the sample. Another example would be to assign each potential subject a number, and then randomly select numbers from a random numbers table to fulfill the required number of subjects for the sample. **Stratified random sampling** is used when the researcher knows some of the variables within a population that will affect the representativeness of the sample. Some examples of variables include age, gender, ethnicity, and medical diagnosis. Thus, subjects are selected randomly on the basis of their classification into the selected stratum. The strata ensure that all levels of the variable(s) are represented in the sample. For example, age could be the variable, and after stratification, the sample might include equal numbers of subjects in the established age ranges of 20–39, 40–59, 60–79, and over 80.

Researchers use **cluster sampling** in two different situations: (1) when the time and travel necessary to use simple random sampling would be prohibitive, and (2) when the specific elements of a population are unknown, therefore making it impossible to develop a sampling frame. In either of these cases, a list of institutions or organizations associated with the elements of interest can often be obtained. To conduct cluster sampling, a list of all the states, cities, institutions, or organizations associated with the elements of the population is developed. The states, cities, institutions, or organizations are then randomly selected from the list to form the sample. Of note is the fact that subjects obtained from the same institution are likely to be somewhat correlated, thus not completely independent (Burns & Grove, 2005). **Systematic sampling** requires an ordered list of all of the members of the population. Individuals are selected through a process that accepts every *k*th member on the list using a randomly selected starting point. *k* is calculated based on the size of population and the sample size desired. For example, if the population has 1,000 potential subjects and a sample size of 100 is desired, then $k = 1,000 \div 100 = 10$. The initial starting point must be random for the sample to be considered a probability sample. Also, steps must be taken to ensure that the original list was not ordered in any way that could affect the study.

Nonprobability Sampling in Quantitative Research

Nonprobability sampling is a nonrandom sampling technique that does not extend equal opportunity for selection to all members of the study population. Readers should never assume a probability sampling method was used; rather, the researchers must identify the sampling method used as probability or nonprobability. Following are descriptions of two common nonprobability sampling methods, convenience and quota, used in quantitative research. Remember that quantitative research is an objective research method used to describe, examine relationships, and determine cause-and-effect interactions among variables (Burns & Grove, 2007). Researchers obtain a **convenience sample** by enrolling subjects who are in the right place at the right time. Subjects are enrolled until the target sample size is obtained. Convenience sampling does not allow for the opportunity to control for biases. To counter the inability to control for biases, researchers must carefully examine the population being studied and adjust the sampling criteria to appropriately include or exclude the identified biases.

Researchers use **quota sampling** to ensure adequate representation of types of subjects who are likely to be underrepresented, such as women, minorities, the elderly, or the poor. A convenience sampling method is used in conjunction with a strategy to ensure the inclusion of the identified subject type. Quota sampling can be used to mimic the known characteristics of the population or to ensure adequate numbers of subjects in each stratum. This is similar to the strategy used for stratified random sampling. Quota sampling is recognized as an improvement over convenience sampling with a decreased opportunity for bias.

Nonprobability Sampling in Qualitative Research

The following sampling methods are still nonprobability sampling methods, meaning that members of the study population do not have equal opportunity to be selected for the sample. These three sampling methods, purposive, network, and theoretical, are more commonly used in qualitative research than quantitative research. Remember that qualitative studies are subjective and are conducted to describe life experiences, cultures, or historical events and give them meaning. **Purposive sampling** occurs when the researcher consciously selects subjects, elements, events, or incidents to include in the study. Those selected by the researchers are information-rich cases, or those from which a lot can be learned. Researchers may make the effort to include typical and atypical cases. This type of sampling has been criticized because the researcher's judgments in the selection of cases cannot be evaluated. However, this sampling method can be a good way to explore new areas of study.

Network sampling makes use of social networks and the fact that friends often have common characteristics. The researcher identifies a few subjects who meet the sampling criteria and then asks them to assist in recruiting others with similar characteristics. Network sampling is sometimes referred to as "snowballing," and is useful for obtaining samples that are difficult to obtain or have not been previously identified for study. Biases are inherent in networking samples since the study subjects are not independent of one another. **Theoretical sampling** is used in the research process to advance the development of a theory. Data are gathered from individuals or groups who can provide relevant information for theory generation. For example, a researcher might interview family members and patients to develop a theory of surviving a near-death experience. The researcher continues to seek subjects and data until saturation of the theory concepts and relationships has occurred. Subject diversity in the sample is promoted to ensure that the developed theory is applicable to a wide range of behaviors and settings (Burns & Grove, 2005).

■ STUDY QUESTIONS

Directions: For each of the following research article excerpts, (1) decide whether the sampling method presented is either a probability or nonprobability sampling method; (2) identify the specific sampling method used, which might include convenience, quota, purposive, network, or theoretical sampling for nonprobability samples or simple random, stratified random, cluster, or systematic sampling for probability samples; and (3) provide a rationale for the sampling method you selected. Some of the examples might include more than one sampling method to obtain the study sample.

1. Study excerpt: "All registered and enrolled nurses who had patient contact and were employed in the ED [Emergency Department] setting were invited to participate in the study." Crilly, J., Chaboyer, W., & Creedy, D. (2004). Violence towards emergency department nurses by patients. *Accident and Emergency Nursing, 12*(2), 67–73. Excerpt from page 69.

2. Study excerpt: "Participants were recruited from a women's shelter with the help of a colleague as contact person, from church support groups within the community by the researcher who made church members aware of the study and the search for participants, and . . . each participant interviewed suggested the name of a potential new participant." Wright, V. L. (2003). A phenomenological exploration of spirituality among African American women recovering from substance abuse. *Archives of Psychiatric Nursing, 17*(4), 173–85. Excerpt from page 176.

3. Study excerpt: "A cross-sectional study was carried out that included 30 prevalent adult patients from a single PD [Peritoneal Dialysis] center. The sample was randomly selected from the outpatient clinic . . . " Vicente-Martinez, M., Martinez-Ramirez, L., Munoz, R., Avila, M., Ventura, M., Rodriguez, E., Amato, D., & Paniagua, R. (2004). Inflammation in patients on peritoneal dialysis is associated with increased extracellular fluid volume. *Archives of Medical Research, 35*(3), 220–4. Excerpt from page 221.

4. Study excerpt: "Participants were recruited from one middle school and two high schools during general assemblies, homeroom classes, or in other required classes (e.g., physical education) so that no student enrolled in particular courses would be excluded . . . The three schools, located within a large, public school district in Houston, Texas, were selected so that (a) a wide range of socioeconomic strata, (b) a balance of males and females, and (c) a locally representative tri-ethnic sample could be attained." Reyes, L. R., Meininger, J. C., Liehr, P., Chan, W., & Mueller, W. H. (2003). Anger in adolescents: Sex, Ethnicity, Age Differences, and Psychometric Properties. *Nursing Research, 52*(1), 2–11. Excerpt from page 4.

5. Study excerpt: "[T]he parents of 120 children aged 5 to 12 years admitted to one of six South Australian hospitals for elective surgery requiring general anesthesia were approached to participate in this study." Wollin, S. R., Plummer, J. L., Owen, H., Hawkins, R. M. F., Materazzo, F., & Morrison, V. (2004). Anxiety in children having elective surgery. *Journal of Pediatric Nursing, 19*(2), 128–32. Excerpt from page 128.

6. Study excerpt: "Doctors were requested to distribute information packs to women in their care, who fulfilled the inclusion criteria of having a diagnosis of Parkinson's Disease and who were still menstruating. . . . [T]he Research Assistant invited an existing participant to introduce or refer her to another woman who might be willing to take part." Fleming, V., Tolson, D., & Schartau, E. (2004). Changing perceptions of womanhood: Living with Parkinson's disease. *International Journal of Nursing Studies, 41*(5), 515–24. Excerpt from page 516.

7. Study excerpt: "A 2-stage . . . sampling method was used to draw a national sample of nurses working in ICUs. . . . After units in U.S. military installations and territories were excluded, the sampling frame provided by the American Hospital Association listed 5,191 ICUs. Based on a power analysis calculation, a random sample of 421 ICUs was chosen using a systematic interval technique." Binkley, C., Furr, L. A., Carrico, R., & McCurren, C. (2004). Survey of oral care practices in U.S. intensive care units. *American Journal of Infection Control, 32*(3), 161–9. Excerpt from page 163.

8. Study excerpt: "All patients were referred by their GP [General Practitioner] to the researcher (L.T.) who, after obtaining informed consent and taking baseline data, randomized the patients" into the experimental group receiving acupuncture and the comparison group receiving standard care. MacPherson, H., Thorpe, L., Thomas, K., & Campbell, M. (2003). Acupuncture for low back pain: Traditional diagnosis and treatment of 148 patients in a clinical trial. *Complementary Therapies in Medicine, 12*(1), 38–44. Excerpt from page 39.

9. Study excerpt: "Potential participants were recruited from youths seeking health and social services from a street outreach program . . . This age group represented the majority of youths seeking services from this program... Saturation (sufficient or adequate data had been collected to meet the goal of the study [to develop a theory]) was reached at the end of 12 interviews; three additional participants were recruited to verify the findings." Rew, L. (2003). A theory of taking care of oneself grounded in experiences of homeless youth. *Nursing Research, 52*(4), 234–41. Excerpt from page 235.

10. Study excerpt: "This study recruited a . . . sample of HIV-positive participants from an Internet Website sponsored by the University of California, San Francisco... as well as HIV-positive patients from five geographic data collection clinical sites located in Boston, MA; New York, NY; Oslo, Norway; Paterson, NJ; and the San Francisco Bay Area from July 1999 to February 2000" and invited them to participate in the study. Chou, F. Y., Holzemer, W. L., Portillo, C. J., & Slaughter, R. (2004). Self-care strategies and sources of information for HIV/AIDS symptom management. *Nursing Research, 53*(5), 332–9. Excerpt from page 333.

ANSWERS TO STUDY QUESTIONS

1. Nonprobability, convenience sampling method. The key is that all the participants were invited to participate in the study. Recall that with convenience sampling, subjects are recruited because they happen to be in the right place at the right time and are invited to participate in a study.

2. Nonprobability, convenience and network sampling methods. Those subjects recruited from the women's shelter and the church support groups were obtained by a sample of convenience. Those subjects were interviewed and asked to suggest the names of other potential subjects, which is network sampling. Network sampling is used by researchers on the basis that members of social sets have similar characteristics.

3. Probability, simple random sampling method. The excerpt states that the subjects were randomly selected. The most common form of probability sampling is simple random sampling.

4. Nonprobability, quota sampling method. The strata identified in this example of quota sampling are socioeconomic status, gender, and ethnicity. Quota sampling is used by researchers to ensure adequate representation by types of subjects that are likely to be underrepresented. This excerpt is not an example of stratified random sampling method because the students were recruited from selected schools and asked to participate, which is convenience sampling. The students were not randomly selected then stratified as is needed for stratified random sampling. The subjects were obtained by a sample of convenience and then organized into strata (socioeconomic status, gender, and ethnicity), which is consistent with the quota sampling method.

5. Nonprobability, convenience sampling method. The participants were admitted to one of six hospitals and asked to participate in the study.

6. Nonprobability, convenience and network sampling methods. The distribution of packets by the doctors to women in their practices represents the convenience sampling method. Participants were invited by the Research Assistant to refer someone else who may be a willing participant, which is network sampling.

7. Probability, cluster and systematic sampling methods. The identification of the sampling frame of ICUs that include the nurses desired for the sample was done using cluster sampling. The sample of 421 ICUs was chosen using a systematic sampling technique. The authors did not describe the interval used during the systematic sampling, but according to the formula given in the discussion of systematic sampling methods, k could be calculated. Thus, $k = 5,191 \div 421 = 12.33$, or every 12th ICU was systematically selected from a random starting point to be included in the study.

8. Nonprobability, convenience sampling method. The subjects were all referred by their general practitioners. After the sample was selected, the subjects were randomized to the experimental group (acupuncture) and comparison group (standard care). The random assignment to groups is part of the design and not the sampling method.

9. Nonprobability, theoretical sampling method. The researchers sought out those who could give information-rich data for the further explanation of a theory. A total of 12 subjects were recruited to achieve saturation of the data for the theory to be developed.

10. Nonprobability, convenience sampling method. Of note, participants were recruited from five differing geographic areas as well as an Internet website and invited to participate in the study, which is consistent with convenience sampling.

■ EXERCISE 9   Questions to be Graded

Directions: For each of the following excerpts, (1) decide whether the sampling method presented is probability or nonprobability; (2) identify the specific type of nonprobability or probability sampling method used; and (3) provide a rationale for the sampling method you selected. Some of the examples might include more than one sampling method to obtain the study sample.

1. Study excerpt: "The sample for this study included 27 Chinese immigrant elders, 11 adult children who were caregivers for Chinese parents, and 12 health and social service providers who served this immigrant group.... Elders were initially recruited through two social service agencies that target Chinese elders in the greater Boston area.... Providers from various disciplines and practice areas were identified by case workers at two social service agencies.... People already participating in the study were asked to refer elders who were not using services at the two initial recruitment sites." Aroian, K. J., Wu, B., & Tran, T. V. (2005). Health care and social service use among Chinese immigrant elders. *Research in Nursing & Health, 28*(2), 95–105. Excerpt from page 97.

2. Study excerpt: "Subjects were recruited through advertisements placed in various newspapers in Lexington, Kentucky.... Individuals reporting any past or present drug- or alcohol-related problems, serious head injuries, learning disabilities, or psychotic symptomatology were excluded from participation." Giancola, P. R. (2004). Difficult temperament, acute alcohol intoxication, and aggressive behavior. *Drug and Alcohol Dependence, 74*(2), 135–45. Excerpt from page 136.

3. Study excerpt: "A mailing list comprising 3,500 randomly selected names and addresses of the 68,000 AACN [American Association of Critical Care Nurses] members was purchased. Every seventh nurse was . . . sampled to yield a group of 500 nurses, all of whom were invited by mail to participate in the study. Two hundred and forty-seven nurses consented to participate (49% response rate) and completed the surveys." Ruggiero, J. S. (2003). Correlates of fatigue in critical care nurses. *Research in Nursing & Health, 26*(6), 434–44. Excerpt from page 437.

4. Study excerpt: "In brief, women 18–35 years old were randomly sampled from census blocks located within a 0.5–miles radius of drug copping sites (sites where crack, cocaine, or heroine are sold)." Alegria, M., Vera, M., Shrout, P., Canino, G., Lai, S., Albizu, C., Marin, H., Pena, M., & Rusch, D. (2004). Understanding hardcore drug use among urban Puerto Rican women in high-risk neighborhoods. *Addictive Behaviors, 29*(4), 643–64. Excerpt from page 645.

5. Study excerpt: "Every weekday, the team selected a minimum of five patients among patients admitted during the preceding 24 h[ours], by a random numbers system. . . . After informed consent, the patients were stratified by age: < or ≥ 60 years, and randomized in blocks of 6, usually sequentially numbered sealed non-transparent envelopes, which were opened to allocate patients into one of two groups: control or intervention." Johansen, N., Kondrup, J., Plum, L. M., Bak, L., Norregaard, P., Bunch, E., Baernthsen, H., Andersen, J. R., Larsen, I. H., & Martinsen, A. (2004). Effect of nutritional support on clinical outcome in patients at nutritional risk. *Clinical Nutrition, 23*(4), 539–50. Excerpt from pages 540-1.

6. Study excerpt: "The 679 subjects who comprise the initial DANDY [Development and Assessment of Nicotine Dependence in Youths] cohort represent a response rate of 94% of the 721 students who were invited, and 76% of all seventh graders (*n* = 900)." DiFranza, J. R., Savageau, J. A., Fletcher, K., Ockene, J. K., Rigotti, N. A., McNeill, A. D., Coleman, M., & Wood, C. (2004). Recollections and repercussions of the first inhaled cigarette. *Addictive Behaviors, 29*(2), 261–72. Excerpt from page 264.

7. Study excerpt: "National lists of NPs [nurse practitioners] and PAs [physician assistants] were obtained from Medical Marketing Services and a total of 3,900 individuals (NPs [*n* = 1,950] and PAs [*n* = 1,950]) were randomly selected from the lists. . . . The stratified samples were assigned randomly in equal allocations to one of three incentive groups." Ulrich, C. M., Danis, M., Koziol, D., Garrett-Mayer, E., Hubbard, R., & Grady, C. (2005). Does it pay to pay? A randomized trial of prepaid financial incentives and lottery incentives in surveys of nonphysician healthcare professionals. *Nursing Research, 54*(3), 178–83. Excerpt from page 179.

8. Study excerpt: "Participants were recruited from a local hospital, a visiting nurse association, a mall health center, and professional referral. . . . Participants were selected to allow diversity of ages, gender, and ethnicity to capture information-rich data that could be used for extrapolation of patterns and themes central to the heart failure experience rather than demographics." Zambroski, C. H. (2003). Qualitative analysis of living with heart failure. *Heart & Lung,* 32(1), 32–40. Excerpt from page 33.

9. Study excerpt: "Participants were recruited through personal acquaintances and professional contacts with several local black ministers . . ." Rodgers, L. S. (2004). Meaning of bereavement among older African American widows. *Geriatric Nursing,* 25(1), 10–16. Excerpt from page 12.

10. Study excerpt: "Patients with baseline [hemoglobin A1c] levels $\geq 7.5\%$ were invited to enroll in the study and assigned randomly to the intervention or control group." Krein, S. L., Klamerus, M. L., Vijan, S., Lee, J. L., Fitzgerald, J. T., Pawlow, A., Reeves, P., & Hawyard, R. A. (2004). Case management for patients with poorly controlled diabetes: A randomized trial. *The American Journal of Medicine,* 116(11), 732–9. Excerpt from page 733.

UNDERSTANDING THE SAMPLING SECTION OF A RESEARCH REPORT: SAMPLE CRITERIA, SAMPLE SIZE, REFUSAL RATE, AND MORTALITY RATE

STATISTICAL TECHNIQUE IN REVIEW

Sampling or eligibility criteria include a list of requirements or characteristics essential for membership in the target population. Sampling criteria include both inclusion and exclusion criteria. **Inclusion sampling criteria** are the requirements identified by the researcher that must be present for an element or subject to be included in a sample. **Exclusion sampling criteria** are the requirements identified by the researcher that eliminate or exclude an element or subject from being in a sample (Burns & Grove, 2007).

The sampling criteria determine the target population, and the sample is selected from the accessible population within the target population. When the study is complete, the researcher hopes to generalize the findings from the sample to the accessible population and then to the target population if the findings are consistent with previous research. A researcher may identify very broad sampling criteria or very specific criteria. The broad sampling criteria can promote a large, diverse, or heterogeneous sample, and the specific sampling criteria promote a smaller, more homogeneous sample (Burns & Grove, 2005).

An adequate sample size is essential for identifying significant relationships among variables or differences between groups. **Power** is the capacity of the study to detect relationships or differences that actually exist in the population. The larger the sample obtained for a study, the greater the power of the study to accurately reject the null hypothesis. The minimum acceptable power for a study is usually set at 0.80 (80%) for research in the health and social sciences.

The researcher needs to identify a large enough accessible population to ensure that an adequate sample is obtained after accounting for refusal and mortality rates. **Refusal rate** is the percentage of potential subjects who decide not to participate in a study. The refusal rate is calculated by dividing the number of potential subjects refusing to participate by the number of potential subjects approached.

$$\text{Refusal rate} = \text{number refusing to participate} \div \text{number of subjects approached} \times 100\%$$

Example: Refusal rate = 5 subjects refusing to participate ÷ 50 subjects approached =
$$5 \div 50 = 0.1 \times 100\% = 10\%$$

Mortality rate is the percent of subjects dropping out of a study for a variety of reasons. Thus, mortality is the loss of subjects after the sample has been selected. The mortality rate is calculated by dividing the number of subjects dropping out of the study by the total number of subjects in the study. Because subject mortality happens for a variety of reasons, researchers must anticipate the mortality rate and increase the number of subjects recruited into a study to ensure an adequate sample size (Burns & Grove, 2007).

Mortality rate = number dropping out of a study ÷ total sample size × 100%
Example: Mortality rate = 4 subjects dropping out of a study ÷ 80 sample size =
4 ÷ 80 = 0.05 × 100% = 5%

The refusal and mortality rates decrease the sample's representativeness of the target population. A refusal rate greater than 10% is of concern, and the researcher needs to determine the impact of this rate on the study findings. In addition, sample mortality also reduces the final sample size and decreases the power of the study to detect relationships among variables and differences between groups. A mortality rate of 10% or greater could impact the ability to accurately reject the null hypothesis in a study. A researcher needs to document the refusal and mortality rates in a study and provide a rationale for both (Burns & Grove, 2007).

RESEARCH ARTICLE

Source: Zeiger, R. S., Bird, S. R., Kaplan, M. S., Schatz, M., Pearlman, D. S., Orav, E. J., Hustad, C. M., & Edelman, J. M. (2005). Short-term and long-term asthma control in patients with mild persistent asthma receiving montelukast or fluticasone: A randomized controlled trial. *The American Journal of Medicine, 118*(6), 649–57.

Introduction

Zeiger et al. (2005) conducted a study "to determine whether montelukast is as effective as fluticasone in controlling mild persistent asthma as determined by rescue-free days. . . . Participants aged 15 to 85 with mild persistent asthma ($n = 400$) were randomized to oral montelukast (10 mg once nightly) or inhaled fluticasone (88 mg twice daily) in a year-long, parallel-group, multi-center study with a 12-week, double-blind period, followed by a 36-week, open-label period. . . . [They found that] the mean percentage of rescue-free days was similar between treatments after 12 weeks . . . but not during the open-label period . . . Although both fluticasone and montelukast significantly improved symptoms, quality of life, and symptom-free days during both treatment periods, greater improvements occurred with fluticasone in lung function during both periods and in asthma control during open-label treatment (Zeiger et al., 2005, p. 649).

Relevant Study Results

"Institutional review boards at each study site ($n = 39$) approved the study protocol, and patients or guardians gave written informed consent. Participants aged 15 to 85 years with symptoms and albuterol use consistent with mild persistent asthma for at least 4 months, as assessed by questionnaire, were recruited. Eligibility criteria were based on National Asthma Education Prevention Program and Global Initiative for Asthma definitions of mild persistent asthma. To ensure a true mild persistent sample, patients were required to meet all of the following criteria: (a) evidence of airway reversibility or hyper-responsiveness documented by at least a 12% increase in FEV_1 [forced expiratory volume] or peak expiratory flow rate after albuterol or a positive methacholine or exercise challenge test; (b) treatment with only as-needed albuterol, (c) an average FEV_1 during the run-in period ≥ 80% of predicted, with none of the qualifying values below 70%; and (d) daytime symptoms and albuterol use on an average of ≥ 2 days, but ≤ 6 days, per week during the 2 weeks before randomization. Patients were excluded if they had used other asthma controller medications or systemic corticosteriods within the past month or required hospital or urgent care for asthma" (Zeiger et al., 2005, p. 650).

"For the 36-week, open-label treatment period, 10% of participants (determined at randomization) switched therapies to preserve the masking in the preceding period. . . . The sample size was determined to provide 90% power with regard to rescue-free days during the double-blind period" (Zeiger et al., 2005, p. 650-1).

"Of the 901 participants screened, 735 entered the placebo run-in period, and 400 were randomized to treatment (Figure 2). The most common reasons for exclusion were asthma being either too mild or too severe. Due to a drug packaging error in which either both active drugs

($n = 11$) or both matching placebos ($n = 9$) were given, 20 randomized participants were discontinued from the study, and their data were excluded from the analyses. Three hundred eighty (380) patients were randomized to masked treatment with montelukast ($n = 189$) or fluticasone ($n = 191$); they were predominantly young, atopic, white, and female. . . . Three hundred fifty participants (92%) completed the double-blind period and continued into the open-label period, and 289 (83%) of these patients completed the study. Reasons for discontinuation are listed in Figure 2" (Zeiger et al., 2005, pp. 651–2).

FIGURE 2 ■ Patient accounting in the MIAMI trial. †As prespecified, 10% of patients (determined at randomization) switched therapies after completing the double-blind period (11 patients from montelukast to fluticasone, 7 patients from fluticasone to montelukast); as a result, the number of patients entering the open-label period in the fluticasone group after the switch was greater than the number of patients in that group who completed the double-blind period. Clinical adverse events leading to patient withdrawal during the double-blind period were asthma (montelukast) and diarrhea, pharyngitis, headache, and insomnia (fluticasone).

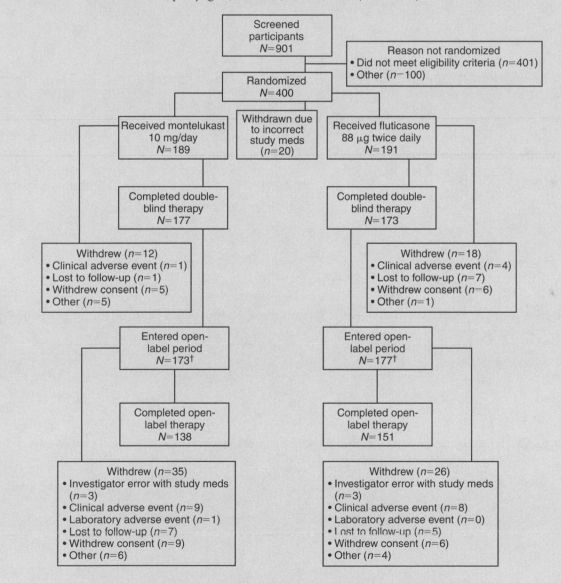

(Zeiger, R. S., Bird, S. R., Kaplan, M. S., Schatz, M., Pearlman, D. S., Orav, E. J., Hustad, C. M., & Edelman, J. M. (2005). Short-term and long-term asthma control in patients with mild persistent asthma receiving montelukast of fluticasone: A randomized controlled trial. *The American Journal of Medicine, 118*(6), p. 652. Copyright © 2005 with permission from Excerpta Medica, Inc.)

■ STUDY QUESTIONS

1. What were the sampling inclusion criteria?

2. How many people met the sampling inclusion criteria and were randomized into groups?

3. How many people completed the research project?

4. What was the sample mortality number? Calculate the mortality rate.

5. Define the term *power* as used in research. What is the minimum power requirement for research? Provide a rationale for your answer.

6. What do the researchers mean by a clinical adverse event, and what were the events in this study?

7. The researchers noted that people withdrew consent at each of the different periods during the MIAMI (Mild Asthma Montelukast versus Inhaled Corticosteroid) trial. Is this sample mortality or refusal rate? Provide a rationale for your answer.

8. If a researcher approached 250 subjects to participate in a study and 230 of these subjects consented to be subjects, what was the refusal rate for this proposed study?

9. Discuss the impact of the refusal rate in Question 8 on the outcome of the study.

ANSWERS TO STUDY QUESTIONS

1. The sample inclusion criteria were "(a) evidence of airway reversibility or hyper-responsiveness documented by at least a 12% increase in FEV_1 [forced expiratory volume] or peak expiratory flow rate after albuterol or a positive methacholine or exercise challenge test, (b) treatment with only as needed albuterol, (c) an average FEV_1 during the run-in period ≥ 80% of predicted, with none of the qualifying values below 70%, and (d) daytime symptoms and albuterol use on an average of ≥ 2 days, but ≤ 6 days, per week during the 2 weeks before randomization"(Zeiger et al., 2005, p. 650).
2. 400 people met the sampling inclusion criteria and were randomized into groups.
3. 289 people completed the research project.
4. Sample mortality rate = number of subjects dropping out of study ÷ sample size × 100%
   Number subjects dropping out of study = 400 sample size – 289 completing study = 111
   Sample mortality rate = 111 subjects dropping out ÷ 400 sample size × 100% = 0.2775 × 100% = 27.75% or 28%
5. Power is the capacity of the study to detect differences or relationships that actually exist in the population. That is, power is the capacity to correctly reject the null hypothesis. The minimum acceptable power is usually set at 0.80 or 80%.
6. Clinical adverse events are problems that are experienced by patients in clinical practice. You have managed these clinical adverse events in your own practice. The clinical adverse events often lead to sample mortality or subjects dropping out of the study. The clinical adverse events causing subjects to withdraw during the double-blind period were asthma, diarrhea, pharyngitis, headache, and insomnia.
7. This is considered part of sample mortality because mortality refers to the loss of subjects from the study after the sample has been selected and the study is being conducted.
8. Refusal rate = number of potential subjects refusing ÷ number of subjects approached × 100%
   Number subjects refusing = 250 – 230 = 20
   Refusal rate = 20 subjects ÷ 250 subjects approached × 100% = 0.08 × 100% = 8%
9. The refusal rate in Question 8 was 8%, which is limited and less than 10% of the subjects approached. Thus, the final sample is probably fairly representative of the accessible population (Burns & Grove, 2005). However, the researcher needs to document the rationale for subjects refusing to participate and determine if there is a trend or specific reason(s) for refusal that might affect the study findings.

■ EXERCISE 10   Questions to be Graded

1. What were the sampling exclusion criteria for the Zeiger et al. (2005) study?

2. Why do you think that the researchers screened 901 patients for their study?

3. Of the 400 subjects randomized to the two treatment groups, what number of participants were discontinued from the study due to a drug packaging error resulting in incorrect study medications? This resulted in what mortality rate for the study?

4. Of the 191 subjects in the fluticasone treatment group, 151 completed the open-label therapy. How many subjects dropped out of this group, and what was the mortality rate from this group during the study? Round your answer to the nearest whole percentage.

5. Discuss the mortality rate in Question 4. Did this mortality rate have a potential effect on the results of this study? Provide a rationale for your answer.

6. The researchers acknowledged that 901 potential subjects were screened and 401 did not meet sample criteria, leaving 500 subjects to be approached for inclusion in this study. Of the 500 potential subjects, 100 were not randomized into groups for "Other" reasons. Assuming that these 100 potential subjects refused to participate in the study, what is the refusal rate for this study? Round your answer to the nearest whole percentage.

7. Do you think that it would have been helpful if the researchers had discussed reasons for refusal? Provide a rationale for your answer.

8. What reasons for sample mortality were provided for this study?

9. Did the sample size provide enough power to correctly reject the null hypothesis with regard to rescue-free days during the double-blind period? Provide a rationale for your answer.

10. Why do you think that it is important for pharmaceutical or drug studies, such as this one, to have a large sample?

EXERCISE

11

USING STATISTICS TO DESCRIBE A STUDY SAMPLE

STATISTICAL TECHNIQUE IN REVIEW

Most studies describe the subjects that comprise the study sample. This description of the sample is called the **sample characteristics** which may be presented in a table or the narrative of the article. The sample characteristics are often presented for each of the groups in a study (i.e. experimental and control groups). Descriptive statistics are used to generate sample characteristics, and the type of statistic used depends on the level of measurement of the demographic variables included in a study (Burns & Grove, 2007). For example, measuring gender produces nominal level data that can be described using frequencies, percentages, and mode. Measuring educational level usually produces ordinal data that can be described using frequencies, percentages, mode, median, and range. Obtaining each subject's specific age is an example of ratio data that can be described using mean, range, and standard deviation. Interval and ratio data are analyzed with the same type of statistics and are usually referred to as interval/ratio level data in this text.

RESEARCH ARTICLE

 Source: Troy, N. W., & Dalgas-Pelish, P. (2003). The effectiveness of a self-care intervention for the management of postpartum fatigue. *Applied Nursing Research, 16*(1), 38–45.

Introduction

Troy and Dalgas-Pelish (2003) conducted a quasi-experimental study to determine the effectiveness of a self-care intervention (Tiredness Management Guide [TMG]) on postpartum fatigue. The study subjects included 68 primiparous mothers, who were randomly assigned to either the experimental group (32 subjects) or the control group (36 subjects) using a computer program. The results of the study indicated that the TMG was effective in reducing levels of morning postpartum fatigue from the 2nd to 4th weeks postpartum. These researchers recommend that "mothers need to be informed that they will probably experience postpartum fatigue and be taught to assess and manage this phenomenon" (Troy & Dalgas-Pelish, 2003, pp. 44-5).

Relevant Study Results

"A total of 80 women were initially enrolled [in the study] . . . twelve of these women dropped out of the study resulting in a final sample of 68." (Troy & Dalgas-Pelish, 2003, p. 39). The researchers presented the characteristics of their sample in a table format for the experimental and control groups (see Table 1). The researchers found no significant differences between the control and experimental groups for any of the demographic or attribute variables.

TABLE 1 ■ Sample Characteristics by Group

Variable	EXPERIMENTAL GROUP			CONTROL GROUP		
	n	*M*	*SD*	*N*	*M*	*SD*
Age (yrs)	32	26.72	5.05	35	26.89	5.25
Income (annual)($)	30	$35,675	$23,969	34	$41,450	$17,527
Length of labor (hrs)	30	14.63	7.78	33	12.79	7.2
Return to work (wks)	8	5.0	1.41	9	5.78	.67
Number of hours working per week	8	34.25	9.15	9	36.68	7.02
	n	%		*n*	%	
Race						
White	23	92		28	96.55	
Black	1	4		0		
Interracial	1	4		0		
Middle Eastern	0			1	3.45	
Marital status						
Married	25	78.1		31	86.1	
Separated/divorced	1	3.1		1	2.8	
Single	6	18.8		3	8.3	
Education						
High school	7	21.9		6	16.7	
Some college	11	34.4		15	41.7	
College graduate or higher	14	43.8		13	36.2	
Type of feeding						
Breast	13	40.6		15	41.7	
Bottle	17	53.1		18	50.0	
Both breast and bottle	2	6.3		2	5.6	
Amount of household and infant care responsibilities						
All	2	6.3		4	11.1	
Most	23	71.9		22	61.1	
One half	5	15.6		7	19.4	
None	1	3.1		0		

Note: Numbers do not always total 32 for experimental group or 36 for control group because of missing data. The percentages do not always total 100% because of missing data.
Troy, N. W., & Dalgas-Pelish, P. (2003). The effectiveness of a self-care intervention for the management of postpartum fatigue. *Applied Nursing Research, 16*(1), p. 40.

■ STUDY QUESTIONS

1. What demographic variables were included in this study?

2. Which of the demographic variables provided ordinal level data? Provide a rationale for your answer.

3. What level of measurement is the data for race?

4. What statistics were used to describe race in this study? Were these appropriate?

5. Could a mean be calculated on the race data? Provide a rationale for your answer.

6. Describe the race of both the experimental and control groups. What does this tell you about the population of this study?

7. What statistics were used to describe age in this study? Were these appropriate? Provide a rationale for your answer.

8. Were the groups similar in age? Provide a rationale for your answer.

9. What was the mode for the type of feeding provided by the experimental and the control groups? Is this mode what you would have expected?

10. Did the experimental group earn similar income to the control group? Provide a rationale for your answer.

ANSWERS TO STUDY QUESTIONS

1. Demographic variables described in the study were: age, income, length of labor, return to work, number of hours working per week, race, marital status, education, type of feeding, and amount of household and infant care responsibilities.

2. The variables education and amount of household and infant care responsibilities are both measured at the ordinal level since the data for each is sorted into categories that can be rank ordered. With education, high school is the lowest level of education, some college is the next level of education, and college graduate or higher is the highest level of education. Care responsibilities include ordinal data that are ranked from a low of "None" to a high of "All."

3. The data collected for race is nominal level since race was measured using mutually exclusive categories of White, Black, Interracial, and Middle Eastern that cannot be rank ordered.

4. Frequencies and percentages were used to describe race for the experimental and control groups. Since the data are nominal, frequencies and percentages were appropriate. The researchers might have also identified the mode, which was White.

5. No, a mean cannot be calculated on the race data. A mean can only be calculated on interval and ratio level data that have numerically equal distances between intervals and not on nominal level data that can only be organized into categories. (See Exercises 1, 2, and 3, which are focused on identifying the level of measurements.)

6. Both the experimental and control groups are predominantly White, 92% and 96.55%, respectively. Thus, the sample is predominately White, and the results are reflective of a White or Caucasian population and not Black, Interracial, or Middle Eastern populations.

7. Age was described for both the experimental and control groups using means and standard deviations. The exact age of the subjects was obtained, providing ratio level data that are descriptively analyzed with means and standard deviations. The researchers might have also provided the range for age for both experimental and control groups.

8. The groups were very similar in age since the mean age for the experimental group was 26.72 and the mean age for the control group was 26.89. The distribution of the ages for the experimental and control groups were also very similar, with standard deviation of 5.05 for the experimental group and 5.25 for the control group.

9. Bottle-feeding was the mode for the experimental (53.1%) and the control (50%) groups since it was the most frequent type of feeding used by both groups. Either a "no" or "yes" answer is correct here as long as you provide a rationale. No, one might expect the mode to be breastfeeding since these were first-time mothers (primiparous) and breastfeeding has such positive outcomes for both infant and mother. Yes, one might expect bottle-feeding to be the mode since many of these mothers planned on returning to work.

10. No, the incomes were not similar for the two groups, but nor was the income significantly different for the groups. The means (M) and standard deviations (SD) for income indicate that the experimental ($M = \$35,675$; $SD = \$23,969$) and control groups ($M = \$41,450$; $SD = \$17,527$) were different. The control group subjects had an M, or mean, that was \$5,775 higher than the experimental group, and the SD was much higher (\$6,442) for the experimental group, indicating a larger range of incomes for that group. However, the narrative from the study indicated that the groups were not significantly different for any of the demographic variables.

Name: _____ Class: _____

Date: _____

■ EXERCISE 11　Questions to be Graded

1. What demographic variables were measured at least at the interval level of measurement?

2. What statistics were used to describe the length of labor in this study? Were these appropriate?

3. What other statistic could have been used to describe the length of labor? Provide a rationale for your answer.

4. Were the distributions of scores similar for the experimental and control groups for the length of labor? Provide a rationale for your answer.

5. Were the experimental and control groups similar in their type of feeding? Provide a rationale for your answer.

6. What was the marital status mode for the subjects in the experimental and control groups? Provide both the frequency and percentage for the marital status mode for both groups.

7. Could a median be determined for the education data? If so, what would the median be for education for the experimental and the control groups? Provide a rationale for your answer.

8. Can the findings from this study be generalized to Black women? Provide a rationale for your answer.

9. If there were 32 subjects in the experimental group and 36 subjects in the control group, why is the income data only reported for 30 subjects in the experimental group and 34 subjects in the control group?

10. Was the sample for this study adequately described? Provide a rationale for your answer.

12 USING POWER ANALYSIS TO DETERMINE SAMPLE SIZE

STATISTICAL TECHNIQUE IN REVIEW

The deciding factor in determining an adequate sample size for descriptive, correlational, quasi-experimental, and experimental studies is power. **Power** is the capacity of the study to detect differences or relationships that actually exist in the population. Expressed another way, power is the capacity to correctly reject the null hypothesis and avoid making a **Type II error**, or saying that the results were nonsignificant when they were significant. When significant results are obtained during a study, then a Type II error has not occurred and the sample size was adequate. The minimum acceptable power for a study is 0.80 or 80%. If a researcher does not have sufficient power to detect differences or relationships that exist in the population, one might question the advisability of conducting the study.

Determining the sample size needed to obtain sufficient power for a study is done by conducting a power analysis. The four elements of **power analysis** are (1) significance level or alpha (α), (2) effect size, (3) power (standard of 0.80 or 80%), and (4) sample size. If three of the four are known, the fourth can be calculated by using power analysis formulas or tables. The **level of significance, or α**, is set by the researcher at the start of the study and is the probability of making a **Type I error**, which is saying results are significant when they are not. The significance level is often set at $\alpha = 0.05$, 0.01, or 0.001, and with $\alpha = 0.05$ there are 5 chances in 100 of making a Type I error. **Effect size (ES)** is the degree to which the null hypothesis is false, or the degree of difference between two groups and the strength of relationships among variables. The ES strengths in studies are commonly labeled as weak, moderate, or strong, where < 0.3 is a weak ES, 0.3–0.5 a moderate ES, and >0.5 a strong ES. These are absolute values since the ES can be positive or negative based on the relationships and differences between groups means found in studies. The anticipated (or expected) ES used to calculate the sample size and power for a planned study is determined from previous research if it exists or is set at a weak or low level of 0.2 or 0.3 for new areas of study (Burns & Grove, 2007). Based on knowing the study alpha, ES, and standard power of 0.80, the researcher can predict the sample size needed for a study.

The adequacy of a study's sample size must be carefully evaluated before data collection. Studies with inadequate sample sizes should not be approved for data collection unless they are the preliminary pilot studies before a planned larger study. Larger sample sizes are difficult to obtain for most health care studies. They require long data-collection periods that are usually very costly. Therefore, the researcher must evaluate the elements of the methodology that affect the required sample size, which include:

1. The more stringent the significance level (e.g. $\alpha = 0.001$ versus $\alpha = 0.05$), the greater the necessary sample size due to the reduced probability of a Type I error. With $\alpha = 0.001$, the probability of error is 1 chance in 1,000; with $\alpha = 0.05$, there are 5 chances for error in 100 studies conducted.

2. Two-tailed statistical tests require larger sample sizes than one-tailed tests.
3. The smaller the effect size, the larger the necessary sample size since the *ES* indicates how strong the relationship is between variables and the strength of the differences between groups.
4. The larger the power required, the larger the necessary sample size.
5. The smaller the sample size, the smaller the power of the study (Burns & Grove, 2005).

RESEARCH ARTICLE 1

Source: Ramey, S. L. (2005). Assessment of health perception, spirituality, and prevalence of cardiovascular disease risk factors within a private college cohort. *Pediatric Nursing, 31*(3), 222–31.

Introduction

Ramey (2005) conducted a study to assess the health perception, spirituality, and prevalence of cardiovascular disease risk factors within a private college cohort. Today's college students are at risk for emotional as well as physical morbidities, and stress appears to be a prevalent factor associated with perceived health. Research has shown that 21% of the college students were overweight, 29% had hypercholesterolemia, and 10% had hypertension. In addition, "more than 12% of the students self-reported feeling so depressed that they could not function on 3-8 occasions last year. Furthermore, 11% of female and 9% of male students were seriously considering suicide on one or more occasions.

Students identified the following as determinants to emotional well-being and impediments to academic success: (1) stress, (2) sleep difficulties, (3) concern for family and friends, and (4) relationship difficulties" (Ramey, 2005, p. 222). Thus, the outcomes of this study might be used to develop strategies to improve the overall health of college community members while considering the unique aspects of this target community.

Relevant Study Results

"Potential subjects were the 644 members of a small private college in Iowa. Surveys were distributed via campus mail, at college meetings, and by direct mail to the neighbors (*n* = 72) living adjacent to the college. Results of the study are based on the percentage of the subjects who returned survey questionnaires (i.e., 62%; *n* = 402 [staff, *n* = 66; faculty, *n* = 72; students, *n* = 287; administrators, *n* = 5; and community, *n* = 17]). . . . Subjects were considered to have provided informed consent by completing and returning the written survey. The study was approved by the research subject's review board" (Ramey, 2005, p. 223).

Ramsey (2005) conducted a power analysis to estimate the sample size needed in her study to prevent a Type II error. The effect size for the study was *ES* = 0.20 and alpha was set at 0.05. Thus, approximately 244 surveys were necessary for data analysis.

■ STUDY QUESTIONS

1. What is the minimum power desired for conducting a study to identify group differences and relationships among variables?

2. What does power mean?

3. Is power analysis conducted to reduce the risk of a Type I or Type II error? If the standard power of 80% or 0.80 is set, what is the chance for error in this study? Provide a rationale for your answer.

4. What are the four elements of power analysis?

5. Did Ramey (2005) have a large enough sample size to detect group differences or relationships among variables in her study? Provide a rationale for your answer.

6. What element of power analysis did the researcher not include in her study? Why do you think this element was omitted from the study?

7. What was the effect size used in this study? What was the strength of this effect size? Why do you think this effect size was used in this study?

8. If the effect size for a study was weak at < 0.3, would a small or large sample be needed to detect significant differences or relationships? Provide a rationale for your answer.

ANSWERS TO STUDY QUESTIONS

1. A minimum power level of 80% (0.80) is desired for conducting a study.
2. Power is the capacity of the study to detect differences or relationships that actually exist in the population. Expressed another way, power is the capacity to correctly reject the null hypothesis and avoid making a Type II error.
3. A power analysis is conducted to reduce the risk of a Type II error, which is when the results were identified as nonsignificant when they were actually significant. With a reduction in the risk for Type II error, the results are more likely to be an accurate reflection of reality and the null hypothesis will be accurately rejected. When power is set at 80%, then the possible error is 0.20 or 20% or 100% − 80% = 20%.
4. The four elements of power are (1) significance level or α, (2) effect size, (3) power, and (4) sample size.
5. Yes, the researcher stated that the power analysis indicated that a sample size of 244 was needed for the study with a power of 0.80 and an $ES = 0.20$. The study included 402 subjects in the sample, so the sample size was adequate for this study to detect group differences or relationships among study variables.
6. The researcher did not state that the power was set at 0.8 or 80%. The power was probably omitted since the standard power of 80% is commonly used to conduct a power analysis. However, it would have been better for the researcher to indicate that the study power was at the standard of 80%, and this would be even more important to state if the power of the study was greater than 80%.
7. The $ES = 0.20$ for this study, which is a weak effect size since it is <0.3 (Burns & Grove, 2007). The weak effect size of 0.20 was probably set in this descriptive study since this was a relatively new area of research and there were inadequate previous studies to determine an ES, or it was calculated from previous studies at 0.20.
8. When the effect size is weak or < 0.3, a large sample is needed to detect significant differences or relationships. The effect size indicates the degree of difference between groups or the strength of relationships among variables. If the difference is small between groups or the relationships among variables are weak, then the effect size is weak, and it takes a larger sample to detect differences and relationships.

RESEARCH ARTICLE 2

Source: Voss, J. A., Good, M., Yates, B., Baun, M. M., Thompson, A., & Hertzog, M. (2004). Sedative music reduces anxiety and pain during chair rest after open-heart surgery. *Pain, 112*(1–2), 197–203.

Introduction

Voss et al. (2004) conducted a study to determine the "effectiveness of non-pharmacological complementary methods (sedative music and scheduled rest) in reducing anxiety and pain [sensation and distress] during chair rest" (Voss et al., 2004, p. 197) after open-heart surgery. The subjects receiving the treatment of sedative music had significantly less anxiety, pain sensation, and pain distress than those subjects in the scheduled rest and the standard care group. The researchers recommend the use of sedative music as an adjuvant to medication for management of anxiety and pain in postoperative patients. The study only involved patients who had had open-heart surgery, which limits the generalization of the findings. Future research is needed to test the effects of music on the anxiety and pain of different types of patients. In addition, research is needed to determine the optimal length for the music sessions and the effectiveness of repeat music sessions in reducing anxiety and pain.

Relevant Study Results

"An experimental, pretest and posttest three-group design was used for this randomized clinical trial. A convenience sample of 62 patients was obtained from a surgical intensive care unit at a rural midwestern hospital over a period of 6 months in 2002. . . . The planned sample size of 96 patients (30 per group plus 6 for attrition) was based on power analysis with an estimated medium effect size of 0.33, power 0.80, alpha = 0.05 and repeated measures analysis of variance. However, preliminary analyses after 62 patients were enrolled revealed significant group differences and large effect sizes for anxiety, pain sensation, and pain distress; thus the data collection was concluded" (Voss et al., 2004, p. 198).

■ EXERCISE 12   Questions to be Graded

1. How large a sample was needed for the Voss et al. (2004) study according to the power analysis? Was this the minimum sample size needed for the study, or did the researchers allow for sample mortality?

2. What was the sample size for the Voss et al. (2004) study? Was this sample size adequate for this study? Provide a rationale for your answer.

3. What effect size was used in conducting the power analysis for this study? What effect size was found during data analysis, and how did this affect the sample size needed for this study?

4. What power was used to conduct the power analysis in the Voss et al. (2004) study? What amount of error exists with this power level? Provide a rationale for your answer.

5. If researchers set the power at 90% to conduct their power analysis, would there be less or more chance of a Type II error than setting the power at 80%? Provide a rationale for your answer.

6. If researchers set the alpha (α) for their study at 0.001 versus 0.05, would they need a smaller or larger sample size? Provide a rationale for your answer.

7. In the discussion section of the research article, the authors stated that sedative music had a large effect size when compared to both usual chair rest (>1.0) and scheduled chair rest (>0.9). Furthermore, scheduled chair rest when compared with usual chair rest did not result in significantly less anxiety, pain sensation, or pain distress, but the differences were in the expected direction with small to medium effects (0.20 to 0.45). Why is this information important for future research?

8. Based on the information provided in Question 7, what effect size(s) would researchers use in conducting a similar study? Provide a rationale for your answer.

9. If a researcher conducted a two-tailed *t*-test versus a one-tailed *t*-test, would they need a smaller or larger sample size? Provide a rationale for your answer.

10. Should the findings from the Voss et al. (2004) study be used in clinical practice? Provide a rationale for your answer.

13

UNDERSTANDING RELIABILITY VALUES OF MEASUREMENT METHODS

STATISTICAL TECHNIQUE IN REVIEW

A **measurement tool is reliable** if it consistently provides the same results every time a specific situation or variable is measured. Two of the most common types of reliability testing include homogeneity and stability. **Homogeneity** testing examines the extent to which all the items in a multiple-item instrument or scale consistently measure a variable. Thus, the internal consistency of a scale is determined with homogeneity testing. **Stability** is concerned with the consistency of repeated measures of the same variable or attribute with the same scale or measurement method over time. Stability is commonly referred to as test-retest reliability due to the repeated measurement of a variable. Reliability testing examines the amount of random error in a measurement technique, and a quality measurement method should have strong reliability. The amount of random error determines the dependability, consistency, and comparability of a measurement method for a study (Burns & Grove, 2005).

Homogeneity or internal consistency of a scale is commonly tested with the Cronbach alpha coefficient (r) for interval and ratio data and the Kuder-Richardson formula (K-R 20) for dichotomous or nominal data. Cronbach's alpha is used to examine internal consistency of multi-item scales such as Likert and Semantic Differential scales. Multi-item scales usually include subscales, and internal consistency is determined for these subscales as well as for the entire scale. A Cronbach alpha score of 1.00 equals perfect reliability, whereas a score of 0.00 indicates no scale reliability. A coefficient of 0.80 is usually considered the lowest suitable reliability value for a scale. When a scale is newly developed, it might have a lower reliability of 0.70 or greater; the reliability usually improves over time as the scale is used in studies and refined (Burns & Grove, 2005).

Readability is an essential component of the reliability, as well as validity, of a measurement method. Readability formulas, now a standard part of word-processing software, count the language elements to provide a probable degree of difficulty of comprehending the text. If researchers mention determining the readability of their measurement methods for a study population, this strengthens the reliability and validity of the instruments used in a study. Subjects must be able to understand the items on a scale in order to complete it accurately (Burns & Grove, 2005).

The concepts of reliability and validity (see Exercise 14) should be evaluated together to determine the quality of a measurement method. An instrument that has low reliability values cannot be valid because it is inconsistent in its measurement. However, an instrument can be reliable and not necessarily valid. For example, a Likert scale to measure pain has a Cronbach's alpha of 0.84, but it does not measure the concept of pain in the elderly. The quality of a study's findings depend on the measurement of study variables with reliable and valid measurement methods (Burns & Grove, 2005). The questions in this exercise will help you learn to evaluate the reliability of instruments used in published studies.

■ STUDY QUESTIONS

1. Based on the information found in "Statistical Technique in Review," what statistical technique is most commonly used to determine homogeneity reliability? Provide a rationale for your answer.

2. What are the lowest and highest reliability coefficients for a multi-item scale? What do those values indicate about the strength of the reliability of the scale?

3. What is the highest reliability score possible? Should a scale have reliability that high? Provide a rationale for your answer.

4. What is the lowest acceptable Cronbach's alpha score for a new measurement tool?

5. What is the lowest acceptable Cronbach's alpha score for an established measurement tool that has been used in several studies over at least 10–15 years?

6. How is stability reliability determined in a study?

7. If the Cronbach's alpha value is $r = 0.60$ for an anxiety scale in a study, how great is the error for this scale in the study? Is this acceptable? Provide a rationale for your answer.

RESEARCH ARTICLE 1

Source: Luffy, R., & Grove, S. K. (2003). Examining the validity, reliability, and preference of three pediatric pain measurement tools in African American children. *Pediatric Nursing, 29*(1), 54–9 (p. 57).

Relevant Study Results

In an effort to determine the most effective scale to measure pain in African American children, Luffy and Grove (2003) examined the validity, reliability, and preference of three different pediatric pain measurement tools. The three tools used in the study were the African American Oucher Scale, the Wong-Baker FACES Scale, and the Visual Analog Scale (VAS). Each child chose a painful experience, rated their experience on each of the above scales, and then chose the scale they liked best. This process was repeated to yield two results, and validity was determined by comparing the rank order of these two painful experiences.

TABLE 1 ■ Overall Preference, Validity, and Reliability for Three Pediatric Pain Intensity Assessment Tools				
	FACES	VAS	Oucher	X^2
Preference	56% (1)	18% (3)	26% (2)	24.08** (**$p < .0001$)
Validity	70% (1)	61% (2)	70% (1)	0.81
Adjusted reliability +	67% (2)	45% (3)	70% (1)	6.12* (*$p < .05$)

Luffy, R., & Grove, S. K. (2003). Examining the validity, reliability, and preference of three pediatric pain measurement tools in African American children. *Pediatric Nursing, 29*(1), 54–9 (p. 57). Reprinted with permission of the publisher, Janetti Publications, Inc., East Holly Avenue, Box 56, Pitman, NJ 08071-0056; 856-256-2300; fax 856-589-7463; www.pediatricnursing.net. For a sample copy of the journal, please contact the publisher.

8. In Table 1, which scale has the highest "Adjusted reliability +"? Which scale has the lowest reliability? What do these results indicate about these scales for this study? Discuss if the scales are reliable in this population.

9. Is there a difference in the "Adjusted reliability +" of the three measurement tools for this sample? Which of the three scales is (are) reliable for this sample? Provide a rationale for your answer.

10. Discuss the importance is having a reliable scale to measure pain in pediatric populations.

■ ANSWERS TO STUDY QUESTIONS

1. The Cronbach's alpha coefficient (r) is calculated to determine the homogeneity or internal consistency of multi-item scales used in research. This r value should be determined for every multi-item scale and its subscales used in a study, since a scale must be reliable for a particular study population in order to obtain useful data from the subjects. Researchers should also discuss the reliability of the scales they use in their study based on previous studies.

2. The range of reliability coefficients can be as low as 0.00 and as high as 1.00, with 0.00 indicating that a measurement method has no reliability or internal consistency in the measurement of a variable, and 1.00 indicating the perfect reliability or consistency of a scale. Negative reliability values can be obtained, but these values indicate a problem with the scale or how the data from the scale were entered in the computer or analyzed.

3. A perfect reliability score is $r = 1.00$ and is the highest possible reliability score for a scale. An $r = 1.00$ is essentially never seen in a study. With perfect reliability, the instrument would be measuring the same thing with the items on a scale, and subjects are giving each item on a scale the same rating. However, it is best when an instrument measures a variety of aspects of a variable and there is variability in the subjects' responses on different items on a scale. For example, if a 20-item tool is measuring depression, then the 20 items should examine different aspects of depression such as depressed mood, loss of appetite, disturbed sleep, and thoughts of harming one's self; and subjects will have different levels of depression that should be identified by a scale. Thus, the reliability value for a scale in a study is best to be less than 1.00 and closer to 0.90.

4. It is best that a scale have a reliability no lower than 0.80. However, a reliability score of 0.70 might be considered an acceptable reliability score for a new scale that will be further revised and refined through research.

5. A reliability score of 0.80 is the lowest acceptable score for an established scale. This means that 80% of the time the scale is reliable or consistent with some chance for random error. The lower the reliability coefficient for a measurement scale, the more error that exists with the scale in measuring a variable in a study.

6. Stability is a type of reliability that is concerned with the consistency of repeated measures of a variable or attribute with the same scale or measurement method over time and is commonly referred to as test-retest reliability. For example if a scale is being used to measure depression in a study, the subjects given this scale should mark the items similarly if they are given the same depression scale two hours apart. If the subjects complete the scale in a similar way from one time to the next, this indicates test-retest reliability.

7. If the Cronbach's alpha coefficient is $r = 0.60$, then the scale has 60% reliability or internal consistency and a high potential for error. It is unacceptable for a scale to have a reliability less than 0.80 or 80% reliability within a study. The researcher cannot trust the data that they have obtained with a scale that has 0.60 reliability. Also if a tool is not reliable, it is not valid.

8. The Oucher scale has the highest "Adjusted Reliability" at 70%. This indicates that the internal consistency or reliability of the Oucher scale in this study is 70%. This is the lowest acceptable reliability value for a new scale that is being refined through additional research. The VAS has the lowest "Adjusted Reliability" at 45% and has a high chance for error. The VAS was not reliable in this population for this study.

9. Yes, there is a difference in the reliability of the three measurement tools. Reliability was 67% for the FACES scale, 45% for the VAS scale, and 70% for the African American Oucher. The Oucher, at 70% reliability, is the scale that is most consistent in the measurement of pain in this pediatric population. The VAS had 45% reliability and the FACES scale has 67% reliability, so these scales were not very reliable in measuring pain in this pediatric population. In addition, the chi square value ($X^2 = 6.12$) is significant at $p < 0.05$, indicating that there is a significant difference among the reliability values for the three tools.

10. A reliable scale is needed to assess pain in a pediatric patient, so the health care providers have consistent and useful information about their patients' pain. The scale needs to provide quality data that can be used to diagnose and effectively manage pain in African American children.

■ EXERCISE 13   Questions to be Graded

RESEARCH ARTICLE 2 FOR QUESTIONS 1-5

 Source: Ashmore, J. A., Emery, C. F., Hauck, E. R., & MacIntyre, N. R. (2005). Marital adjustment among patients with chronic obstructive pulmonary disease who are participating in pulmonary rehabilitation. *Heart & Lung, 34*(4), 270–8.

Relevant Study Results

"Psychological well-being was assessed with 4 self-report scales. (1) The State-Trait Anxiety Inventory is a 40-item measure of both immediate and longer-standing symptoms of anxiety. . . . Calculation of reliability with the study sample indicated a coefficient alpha of .93. (2) The Center for Epidemiological Studies–Depression Scale is a 20-item measure developed for evaluating depressive symptoms in community-residing older adults. Calculation of reliability with the study sample indicated a coefficient alpha of .89. (3) The Bradburn Affect-Balance Scale is a 10-item scale developed for use with older adults and assesses both positive and negative emotions. Calculation of reliability with the study sample indicated a coefficient alpha of .72. (4) Stress was measured by a self-report scale . . . Calculation of reliability with the study sample indicated a coefficient alpha of .76" (Ashmore et al., 2005, pp. 272–3).

For Questions 1 through 5, please refer to the Relevant Study Results for Research Article 2.

1. Based on the information provided from the Ashmore et al. (2005) study, which scale has the strongest reliability? Provide a rationale for your answer.

2. Based on the information provided from the Ashmore et al. (2005) study, which scale has the weakest reliability? Provide a rationale for your answer.

3. What type of reliability is provided for the four scales used in the Ashmore et al. (2005) study? Provide a rationale for your answer.

4. Are four scales used in the Ashmore et al. (2005) study examined for validity? Provide a rationale for your answer.

5. Are four scales in the Ashmore et al. (2005) study reliable in this study? Provide a rationale for your answer.

RESEARCH ARTICLE 3 FOR QUESTIONS 6-10

Source: Ely, B., Alexander, L. B., & Reed, M. (2005). The working alliance in pediatric chronic disease management: A pilot study of instrument reliability and feasibility. *Journal of Pediatric Nursing, 20*(3), 190–200.

Relevant Study Results

In this study, the researchers examined the reliability of the Working Alliance Inventory for Chronic Care (WAICC) scales (both 12-item and 36-item scales) that were developed to evaluate the alliances among a subject (child or adolescent), the health care providers (MD or NP), and the parent/guardian. "Internal consistency reliability estimates using Cronbach's alpha for the first administration yielded alpha scores ranging from .76 to .88 indicating strong internal consistency [for the WAICC]. Cronbach's alpha scores for the first administration of the 12-item child version of the WAICC were .84 (child's relationship with MD or NP) and .88 (parent perception of their child's relationship with the MD or NP). Using the 36-item scale, alphas ranged from .76 (adolescent's relationship with MD or NP) to .86 (parent perception of their adolescent's relationship with MD or NP). . . . As mentioned previously, test-retest reliability was analyzed using data from initial sample only. . . . Test-retest reliability was stronger in the child participants than for the adolescent participants" (Ely et al., 2005, p. 196).

For Questions 6 through 10, please refer to the Relevant Study Results from Research Article 3.

6. The 36-item WAICC Scale was most reliable for which group? Was this scale reliable for this study? Provide a rationale for your answer.

7. The Cronbach's alpha coefficient was .84 for the 12-item child version of the WAICC for the child's relationship with the MD or NP. What does this value indicate in terms of internal consistency of this scale?

8. The Cronbach's alpha coefficient was .88 for the 12-item child version of the WAICC for the parent's perception of his or her child's relationship with MD or NP. The Cronbach's alpha coefficient is used to determine what type of reliability for a scale? Provide a rationale for your answer.

9. The WAICC Scales were examined using test-retest reliability. What type of reliability is test-retest reliability? Was the test-retest reliability stronger for the adolescent or child participants?

10. Are the 12- and 36-item WAICC scales reliable in the Ely et al. (2005) study? Provide a rationale for your answer.

14 UNDERSTANDING VALIDITY VALUES OF MEASUREMENT METHODS

STATISTICAL TECHNIQUE IN REVIEW

A measurement method has **validity** if it accurately reflects the concept it is supposed to be measuring. In examining validity, you focus on the appropriateness, meaningfulness, and usefulness of a measurement method. For research purposes, the term *validity* is synonymous with the term *construct validity*. **Construct validity** is a single broad evaluation of measurement methods and includes content-related validity, convergent validity, divergent validity, validity from factor analysis, validity from contrasting groups, validity from prediction of concurrent and future events, and successive verification validity.

Content-related validity examines the extent to which the measurement method includes all the major elements relevant to the concept being measured. The major elements to be included in an instrument are determined by a review of literature; construction of the scale based on the literature; and then review by an expert panel for completeness, conciseness, clarity, and readability. Readability of a measurement method is also examined with formulas, which are now a standard part of word-processing software, that count the language elements to provide a probable degree of difficulty of comprehending the text of the instrument. Readability is an essential component of validity as well as reliability since an instrument must be read and understood to be reliable and valid (Burns & Grove, 2005).

Convergent validity is examined by comparing a new instrument with an existing instrument that measures the same concept or construct. The validity of both instruments is strengthened when the two instruments positively correlate at 0.4 or higher. For example, if the data from measuring depression with two scales resulted in a correlation of 0.4 or higher, then the convergent validity of both scales would be strengthened. **Divergent validity** is examined when a new instrument measures another concept or an opposite concept of the existing instrument. For example, two different scales, one measuring hope and the other measuring hopelessness, could be examined for divergent validity. If the two measurement strategies have a negative correlation of –0.4 or stronger, the divergent validity of both scales is strengthened (Burns & Grove, 2005).

Validity from factor analysis examines if an instrument includes the elements of the concept being measured. A researcher uses exploratory and/or confirmatory factor analysis to determine if the items in an instrument are related and cluster together to form factors that reflect the elements of the concept being measured. The factors identified with factor analysis can then be compared with the elements of the concept identified through the review of literature with content-related validity. If the factor analysis results identify the essential elements of the concept to be measured by an instrument, then the validity of the instrument is strengthened (Burns & Grove, 2005).

Validity from contrasting groups is tested by identifying groups that are expected or known to have contrasting scores on an instrument and then asking the groups to complete the instrument.

If the two groups have contrasting scores on the instrument, then the validity of the instrument is strengthened. For example, researchers could compare the scores on a depression scale for a group of patients diagnosed with depression and a group of individuals who do not have a depression diagnosis. If the groups have contrasting scores, then the depression scale is thought to measure the concept of depression and the validity of the scale is strengthened.

Validity from the prediction of future events is achieved when the scores on an instrument can be used to predict future performance or attitudes. For example, a fall risk assessment scale has been developed to predict the fall rate in the elderly. The positive relationship of the scale score with the incidence of falls in the elderly strengthens the validity of this scale to determine the risk for falling. **Validity from prediction of concurrent events** can be tested by examining the ability to predict the concurrent value of one instrument on the basis of the value obtained on an instrument to measure another concept. For example, researchers might use the results from a self-esteem scale to predict the results on a coping scale. Thus, if subjects with high self-esteem scores had high coping scores, then this would add to the validity of the self-esteem scale.

Successive verification validity is achieved when an instrument is used in additional studies with a variety of subjects. Thus, an instrument's validity is strengthened over time with its use in several studies. In summary, there are a variety of ways to add to the validity of an instrument, and the measurement section of a study needs to address the validity of the instruments used in the study. The instrument validity information is often provided from previous research, but sometimes a study might include examining an instrument's validity. The concepts of reliability and validity are usually both evaluated in the measurement section of a research article because an instrument cannot be valid if it is not reliable. An instrument must be both reliable and valid to accurately measure a concept in a study (Burns & Grove, 2005).

■ STUDY QUESTIONS

1. Validity of a measurement method can be developed in several ways. Identify the ways that the construct validity of an instrument can be strengthened.

2. What is the difference between convergent and divergent validity? When is convergent and divergent validity of an instrument strengthened?

3. Can a measurement method be valid if it is not reliable? Provide a rationale for your answer.

4. A measurement method that predicts the rate of pressure ulcer development in hospitalized patients has what type of validity?

5. Which scale would have stronger validity for the measurement of the concept of anxiety: a scale developed five years ago and used frequently in studies, or a scale just developed for a study? Provide a rationale for your answer.

RESEARCH ARTICLE 1

 Source: Luffy, R., & Grove, S. K. (2003). Examining the validity, reliability, and preference of three pediatric pain measurement tools in African American children. *Pediatric Nursing, 29*(1), 54-59.

Relevant Study Results

In an effort to determine the best tool to measure pain in African American children, Luffy and Grove (2003) examined the validity, reliability, and preference of three pediatric pain scales. The scales studied were the African American Oucher Scale, the Wong-Baker FACES Scale, and the Visual Analog Scale (VAS). Each child chose a painful experience, rated their experience on each of the above scales, and then chose the scale they liked best. This process was repeated to yield two results, and validity was determined by comparing the rank order of these two painful experiences.

TABLE 1 ■ Overall Preference, Validity, and Reliability for Three Pediatric Pain Intensity Assessment Scales				
	FACES	VAS	OUCHER	χ^2
Preference	56% (1)	18% (3)	26% (2)	24.08** (**$p \leq$ .0001)
Validity	70% (1)	61% (2)	70% (1)	0.81
Adjusted reliability +	67% (2)	45% (3)	70% (1)	6.12* (*$p <$ .05)

Luffy, R., & Grove, S. K. (2003). Examining the validity, reliability, and preference of three pediatric pain measurement tools in African American children. *Pediatric Nursing, 29*(1), 54–9.

6. In Table 1, is there a difference in the validity of the three scales? If a difference exists, is it statistically significant?

7. In Table 1, what values for preference are listed for each measurement tool? Are these preference values significantly different statistically? Provide a rationale for your answer.

8. Luffy and Grove (2003) addressed pain assessment for African American children and examined the validity, reliability, and preference of subjects from this population. Why do you think the African American children preferred the FACES Scale over the African American Oucher Scale?

9. Based on the information provided in Table 1, what scale would be the best to use in assessing the pain of African American children in clinical practice? Provide a rationale for your answer.

■ ANSWERS TO STUDY QUESTIONS

1. An instrument is considered valid if it measures what it is supposed to measure and validity is synonymous with the term *construct validity*. Construct validity is a single, broad evaluation of measurement methods and includes content-related validity, convergent validity, divergent validity, validity from factor analysis, validity from contrasting groups, validity from prediction of concurrent and future events, and successive verification validity.

2. Convergent validity is examined by determining the relationship between instruments that measure the same concept, such as two scales to measure depression. The correlation should be positive at 0.4 or higher to strengthen the validity of the scales. Divergent validity is examined by comparing the scores from an instrument that measures another or opposite concept from an existing instrument. The correlation should be negative, at least –0.4 or higher, to strengthen the validity of the instruments.

3. A measurement method cannot be valid if it is not reliable. To be reliable, an instrument must consistently measure something. If the instrument cannot consistently measure something, then it cannot provide a valid or accurate measurement of the concept the researcher desires to measure.

4. This is an example of validity from the prediction of future events, where an instrument is used to predict the event of pressure ulcer. The validity of the instrument is strengthened if it can successfully predict an event.

5. The scale developed five years ago to measure anxiety that has been used in a variety of studies with different populations has greater successive verification validity than the scale just developed for a study. Thus, if the scale has been used in other studies, a researcher has a more valid scale to use in a study than a new scale.

6. Validity results were 70% for both the FACES and Oucher scales, and 61% was reported for the VAS. There is no significant difference among the three scales for validity with $\chi^2 = 0.81$.

7. From Table 1, the values for preference are as follows: FACES 56%, VAS 18%, and Oucher Scale 26%. The FACES scale was preferred nearly two times more than the Oucher scale and more than three times the VAS scale. The χ^2 value for preference is 24.08. This value is reported statistically significant at $p \leq 0.0001$, which is extremely significant with minimal chance that the results are an error.

8. Answers may vary. The preference scores indicate that the FACES scale was probably the easiest scale for the children to use and the one they could best relate to when judging the severity of their pain. The literature review in the Luffy and Grove (2003) article indicates that children are less likely to see prejudice and that it does not matter to them that the pictures they are looking at are of children of the same or different race. Thus, the simplest tool, FACES with the drawn happy and sad faces, was more appealing to the children in this study than the African American Oucher Scale.

9. Answers may vary. Based on the reported reliability, validity, and preference scores, the FACES would be the best scale for assessing pain severity in African American pediatric patients. This scale had strong reliability at 67% and the strongest validity at 70%, and it was the most preferred scale by the children. In clinical practice, it is important to have a scale that children prefer to use and that is reliable and valid. If you just examined the validity and the reliability values, then the OUCHER, with the 70% for both validity and reliability, would be considered the strongest measurement method. However, it has such poor preference by the children that it might not be used as readily in clinical practice. When examining reliability, validity, and preference, the FACES has the greatest strength for use in this population.

■ EXERCISE 14 Questions to be Graded

RESEARCH ARTICLE 2

 Source: Dobratz, M. C. (2004). The life closure scale: Additional psychometric testing of a tool to measure psychological adaptation in death and dying. *Research in Nursing & Health, 27*(1), 52–62.

Relevant Study Results

Dobratz developed a Life Closure Scale (LCS) in 1990 to explore the dimensions of psychological adaptation in terminal illness. The focus of this research article was the expansion of the reliability and validity of the LCS (Dobratz, 2004). The following excerpt from this study discusses the quality of LCS as a measure of psychological adaptation in terminal illness.

"The 45-item LCS was designed as a 5-point Likert-type scale with a scaling format that ranges from 1 (a little of the time) to 5 (most of the time), with higher scores indicating increased psychological adaptation.... LCS has two reliable subscales: (1) the self-reconciled and (2) the self-restructuring.... A Cronbach's alpha of .80 was obtained for the total scale, with consistency reliabilities of .85 (self-reconciled) and .86 (self-restructuring) for the subscales.

"Convergent and divergent validity was established with the City of Hope Medical Center Quality of Life (QOL) Survey ... and the Zung Depression Scale.... The total LCS converged with those items in the QOL survey that measured psychological well-being (.82), with the self-restructuring showing a moderate correlation of .69, and the self-reconciled a lower correlation of .37.... [T]he LCS diverged from the Zung subscale of psychological disturbance and showed low negative correlations for self-restructuring (−.46) and self-reconciled (−.38). The total LCS and the Zung subscale of psychological disturbance showed a moderate negative correlation of −.60" (Dobratz, 2004, p. 55). By definition of this author, −.60 is considered a strong negative correlation.

"To assure that the scale's theoretical structure was valid and the correlations between the variables were ordered ... factor analysis was performed on the 20-item LCS" (Dobratz, 2004, p. 56). The factor analysis identified two major variables that were consistent with the two subscales of self-restructuring and self-reconciled.

"The two independent subscales of the ABS [Affect Balance Scale], the Positive Affect Scale (PAS) and the Negative Affect Scale (NAS), were then correlated with the LCS.... A significant correlation between the LCS and the PAS ($r =.36$, $p <.001$) showed a significant and positive relationship between the tool and a measure of psychological well-being. The correlation between the LCS and the NAS was $r = -.59$, $p <.001$), showing a significant negative association of the LCS with mental distress" (Dobratz, 2004, p.57).

For Questions 1 through 7, please refer to the excerpt from Research Article 2.

1. The correlation of the total LCS and its two subscales of self-reconciled and self-restructuring with the Zung Depression Scale is an example of what type of construct validity? Provide a rationale for your answer.

2. Were the correlational values of the Zung Depression Scale with the total LCS and its two subscales acceptable to strengthen the validity of the LCS? Provide a rationale for your answer.

3. The correlation of the total LCS and its two subscales of self-reconciled and self-restructuring with the Quality of Life (QOL) Survey is an example of what type of construct validity? Provide a rationale for your answer.

4. Were the correlational values of the QOL Survey with the total LCS and its two subscales acceptable to strengthen the validity of the LCS? Provide a rationale for your answer.

5. The correlation of the LCS with the NAS is an example of what type of construct validity? Is this correlational value acceptable to strengthen the validity of the LCS? Provide a rationale for your answer.

6. Besides the convergent and divergent validity information, is there any other type of construct validity addressed in the Relevant Study Results of Research Article 2? If so, describe the type of validity.

7. Based on the information provided from the Dobratz (2004) study, do you think the LCS is a quality measurement method with acceptable reliability and validity? Provide a rationale for your answer.

RESEARCH ARTICLE 3

Source: Champion, V., Skinner, C. S., & Menon, U. (2005). Development of a self-efficacy scale for mammography. *Research in Nursing & Health, 28*(4), 329–36.

Relevant Study Results

Champion et al. (2005) developed a self-efficacy scale for mammography. "A Cronbach alpha correlation coefficient of .87 was obtained for the total self-efficacy scale" (Champion et al., 2005, p. 332). Confirmatory factor analysis was conducted on the self-efficacy scale data to determine the theoretical structure of the scale. In addition, the self-efficacy scale was given to subjects to predict the likelihood of women getting a mammogram.

For Questions 8 through 10, please refer to the excerpt from Research Article 3.

8. Using the self-efficacy scale to predict the likelihood of women getting a mammogram is an example of what type of construct validity? Provide a rationale for your answer.

9. Why was confirmatory factor analysis done in this study?

10. Discuss the reliability and validity of the self-efficacy scale. Would you recommend the use of this scale to measure self-efficacy for mammography in your patients?

15

MEASUREMENT OF CENTRAL TENDENCY: MEAN, MEDIAN, AND MODE

STATISTICAL TECHNIQUE IN REVIEW

Mean, median, and mode are the three measures of central tendency used to describe study variables. These measures of central tendency are analysis techniques used to determine the center of a distribution of data, and the central tendency calculated is based on the level of measurement of the data. The **mode** is the most frequently occurring score of a distribution. The mode is the only acceptable measure of central tendency for analyzing nominal level data, which are not numeric and cannot be ranked, compared, or subjected to mathematic operations. If a distribution has two scores that occur more frequently than others, the distribution is called **bimodal**. A distribution with more than two modes is **multimodal**. The **median** *(MD)* is a score that lies in the middle of a rank ordered list of values of a distribution. If a distribution consists of an odd number of scores, the *MD* is the middle score that divides the rest of the distribution into two equal parts. In a distribution with an even number of scores, the *MD* is half of the sum of the two middle numbers of that distribution. If several scores in a distribution are of the same value, then the *MD* will be the value of the middle score. The *MD* is the most precise measure of central tendency for ordinal level data and for non-normally distributed or skewed interval or ratio level data. The following formula can be used to calculate a median in a distribution of scores.

$$\text{Median} = \frac{N + 1}{2}$$

Example: $N = 31$ $\text{Median} = \frac{31 + 1}{2} = 32 \div 2 = 16^{\text{th}}$ score

N is the number of scores

Example: $N = 40$ $\text{Median} = \frac{40 + 1}{2} = 41 \div 2 = 20.5^{\text{th}}$ score

Thus, the median is half way between the 20th and the 21st scores.

The **mean** $(\bar{X})$ is the arithmetic average of all scores of a sample, that is, the sum of its individual scores divided by the total number of scores. The mean is the most accurate measure of central tendency for normally distributed data of interval and ratio levels and can only be used for those levels of data (Burns & Grove, 2005). The formula for the mean is:

$$\text{Mean} = \frac{\Sigma X}{N}$$

ΣX is the sum of the raw scores in a study

N is the sample size or number of scores in the study

Example: Raw scores = 8, 9, 9, 10, 11, 11 $N = 6$ $\text{Mean} = 58 \div 6 = 9.666 = 9.67$

RESEARCH ARTICLE

Source: Happell, B. (2002). The role of nursing education in the perpetuation of inequality. *Nurse Education Today, 22*(8), 632–40.

Introduction

Happell (2002) examined the effect of nursing education on the specialty preferences of under-graduate nursing students in Australia. The students were given a questionnaire asking them to rank nine nursing specialties from 1 = most desirable to 9 = least desirable. The questionnaire was administered at the beginning of the program (stage 1, $n = 793$) and towards its end (stage 2, $n = 521$). The results showed some differences in students' preference of specialty area from the beginning to the end of their educational program, but the influence was limited. Nursing specialties that were initially selected as most favorable, such as pediatrics, midwifery, and critical care, remained popular towards the end of the educational program. In addition, the specialties that were favored the least at the beginning of the educational program, such as gerontology, psychiatric, and community nursing, were still ranked as least desirable towards the end.

Relevant Study Results

"A growing body of literature now strongly supports the view that undergraduate nursing students commence their education program with firm views about the most desirable and undesirable areas of practice. This paper reports the results of a longitudinal study of undergraduate nursing students' career preferences in which attitudes on commencement [of their educational program] are compared to attitudes immediately prior to the completion [of their program]" (Happell, 2002, p. 632). The results suggest that the career preferences of nursing students are not static and have been influenced during the 3 years of nursing education, but the influence is limited. The mean, median, and mode ranking of the nursing specialty areas by the nursing students at the start of their program are presented in Table 1, and the mean, median, and mode ranking of specialty areas at the end of the educational program are presented in Table 2.

TABLE 1 ■ The Relative Popularity of Nursing Specialities Assessed at the Start of the Nursing Course ($n = 793$) Ordered by Mean Ranking				
Rank	Nursing Specialty	Mean Ranking[a]	Median Ranking[a]	Mode of the Ranking[a]
1	Working with children	3.34	3.0	2.0
2	Midwifery	3.77	3.0	1.0
3	Intensive/critical care	3.96	4.0	3.0
4	Operating theatre	3.98	4.0	2.0
5	General surgical nursing	4.92	5.0	5.0
6	General medical nursing	5.02	5.0	6.0
7	Community health nursing	5.85	6.0	7.0
8	Psychiatric nursing	6.92	8.0	9.0
9	Working with the elderly	7.15	8.0	9.0

[a]Rankings are from 1 = most popular to 9 = least popular.
Happell, B. (2002). The role of nursing education in the perpetuation of inequality. *Nurse Education Today, 22*(8), p. 635.

Rank	Nursing Specialty	Mean Ranking[a]	Median Ranking[a]	Mode of the Ranking[a]	Sig. (2-tailed)
	TABLE 2 ■ The Relative Popularity of Nursing Specialties Assessed at the end of the Nursing Course (n = 521) Ordered by Mean Ranking				
1	General surgical nursing	3.90	4	2	.000
2	Intensive/critical care	4.28	4	1	.869
3	Working with children	4.31	4	2	.354
4	Midwifery	4.53	4	1	.045
5	Operating theatre	4.78	5	5	.000
6	Community health nursing	4.78	5	7	.058
7	General medical nursing	4.86	5	5	.081
8	Psychiatric nursing	5.95	7	9	.011
9	Working with the elderly	7.45	8	9	.000

[a]Rankings are from 1 = most popular to 9 = least popular.
Happell, B. (2002). The role of nursing education in the perpetuation of inequality. *Nurse Education Today, 22*(8), p. 635.

"Some notable differences in students' career preferences have occurred [at the end of the educational program (stage 2)] with all of the areas ranked from 1 to 5 being different from those recorded [at the start of the program (stage 1)]. Three of these changes were analyzed as statistically significant. On closer analysis, however, it becomes apparent that the five most popular choices at stage 1 continue to be the five most popular choices at stage 2, with the difference reflecting a change in order" (Happell, 2002, p. 634).

■ STUDY QUESTIONS

1. What is/are the mode(s) of the following pain intensity ratings of 10 postoperative patients who were asked to rate their pain on a 0–10 scale: 3, 4, 5, 4, 3, 3, 8, 2, 4, 9? Is the distribution unimodal, bimodal, or multimodal? Provide a rationale for your answer.

2. Calculate the mean ($\bar{X}$) and the median (*MD*) values for the distribution of the pain intensity scores presented in Question 1.

3. Which measure of central tendency always represents an actual score of the distribution?
   a. Mean
   b. Median
   c. Mode
   d. Range

4. According to Table 1, which nursing specialty was considered to be the most popular career choice among the nursing students at the beginning of their educational program? What rank was this specialty area most frequently assigned?

5. According to data in Table 1, which nursing specialty area was the least popular among the nursing students at the start of their program? Which score was in the middle of the rank ordered distribution of scores assigned to this specialty by the students entering the program?

6. What was the arithmetic average of all ranks assigned to the general medical nursing specialty area by the nursing students entering the program?

7. According to Table 1, working with the elderly and psychiatric nursing had equal median and mode. Which specialty area was more popular? Provide a rationale for your answer.

8. Compare the mean rankings of working with the elderly between Tables 1 and 2. How did the popularity of this specialty among the nursing students change?
   a. Its popularity remained unchanged.
   b. Its popularity increased slightly.
   c. Its popularity decreased slightly.
   d. Its popularity increased greatly.

9. The ranking of which nursing specialty in Table 2 is closest to being normally distributed? Provide a rationale for your answer.

10. Assuming that $\alpha = 0.05$, which nursing specialties have undergone a significant change in popularity between stages 1 and 2 of the research questionnaire administration?

◼ ANSWERS TO STUDY QUESTIONS

1. The set of values describing pain intensity ratings of postoperative patients has two modes or is bimodal. Its two modes, or its most frequently occurring scores, are 3 and 4. Both scores occur in the distribution three times. So, the above distribution of scores is bimodal because it has two scores (3 and 4) that occur more frequently than other scores of the distribution.

2. $\bar{X} = 4.5, MD = 4. \bar{X} = (3 + 4 + 5 + 4 + 3 + 3 + 8 + 2 + 4 + 9) \div 10 = 45 \div 10 = 4.5$. To determine the MD value of the distribution, arrange the pain scores in the order of increasing intensity first: 2, 3, 3, 3, 4, 4, 4, 5, 8, 9. Since this distribution has an even number of values, but the two middle scores are 4, the median is 4.

3. Answer: c. Mode. Mode is the most frequently occurring score of a distribution and thus will always be an actual score of the distribution. Mean is the average of all scores, so it may not be an actual score of the distribution. Median is the middle score of the distribution, which, with an even number of items, may not be an actual score in the distribution. The range is a measure of dispersion and not a measure of central tendency.

4. The most popular career choice of nursing students at the beginning of their educational program was working with children, which is at the top of the list in Table 1. However, the most frequent rank assigned to this specialty, or the mode of all ranks assigned to it, was 2.

5. Working with the elderly was ranked the lowest compared to the other nursing specialty areas. The median, or 8 in this study, was the score that was in the middle of the rank ordered distribution of all scores assigned to this specialty. The median is at the 50% or the middle of the distribution.

6. 5.02 is the mean or arithmetic average for general medical nursing specialty in Table 1.

7. As indicated by its mean ranking of 6.92, psychiatric nursing was a more popular nursing specialty area than working with the elderly, with a mean ranking of 7.15. The lower the mean ranking, the more popular the nursing specialty was in this sample.

8. Answer: c. Its popularity decreased slightly. The mean ranking for working with the elderly was 7.15 at the start of the educational program and 7.45 at the end of the program. Thus, the mean ranking increased from 7.15 to 7.45, showing that a few more students assigned higher (less popular) ranks to this specialty at the end of the program than at the start. The larger the mean ranking, the less popular the specialty area is in this study.

9. In normally distributed data, $\bar{X} = MD = $ mode. The nursing specialty that fits this requirement the best in Table 2 is Medical nursing: mode = median = 5, $\bar{X} = 4.86$, which is almost 5.

10. The results are in Table 2, and surgical nursing, midwifery, operating theatre, psychiatric nursing, and working with the elderly had $p < 0.05$, so all of these nursing specialties had undergone a significant change in popularity from the start to the end of the nursing educational program.

■ EXERCISE 15   Questions to be Graded

1. The following list represents the number of nursing students enrolled in a particular nursing program between the years of 2001 and 2007, respectively: 563, 593, 606, 520, 563, 610, 577. Determine the mean, median, and mode of the number of the nursing students enrolled in the above program between 2001 and 2007. Show your calculations.

2. According to Table 2, which nursing specialty had the rank of 7 as its most frequently assigned rank?

3. According to Table 2, which nursing specialty had an arithmetic average of all its ranks that equaled 4.31?

4. Which nursing specialty was ranked as the second most popular by the nursing students at the time of completion of their program? Which rank represented the 50th percentile of all ranks assigned to that specialty?

5. Which of the following nursing specialties has undergone a significant change in popularity yet retained the same median and mode rankings by the nursing students at the beginning and end of their program?
   a. Medical nursing
   b. Psychiatric nursing
   c. Working with the elderly
   d. Surgical nursing

6. Which nursing specialty demonstrated the most dramatic ascent in both mode ranking and popularity?

7. Based on the information presented in the Relevant Study Results and in Tables 1 and 2, which of the following statements regarding the specialty preferences of the nursing students in this study is true?
   a. Specialty preferences of nursing students are not static.
   b. Nursing education has a significant influence on the career preferences of nursing students.
   c. Specialty preferences of nursing students are static.
   d. Nursing education resulted in a decrease in the popularity of the psychiatric nursing specialty by nursing students.

8. The ranking of which nursing specialty in Table 1 is closest to being normally distributed? Provide a rationale for your answer.

9. Assuming that $\alpha = 0.01$, which nursing specialties demonstrated a significant change in popularity between the stages 1 and 2 of the research questionnaire administration? Provide a rationale for your response.

10. What is the most accurate measure of central tendency for the type of data collected in this study? Provide a rationale for your answer.

16

MEAN AND STANDARD DEVIATION

STATISTICAL TECHNIQUE IN REVIEW

The mean ($\bar{X}$) is a measure of central tendency for a set of data and is the arithmetic average calculated for the data. (Please refer to Exercise 15 for further information about the mean). The **standard deviation** (*SD)* is a measure of dispersion and is the average amount of points by which the scores of a distribution vary from the mean. When the scores of a distribution deviate from the mean considerably, the *SD* or spread of scores is large. When the degree of deviation of scores from the mean is small, the *SD* or spread of the scores is small. Both the $\bar{X}$ and *SD* are descriptive statistics calculated to describe study variables (Burns & Grove, 2007).

RESEARCH ARTICLE

Source: Tsay, S. L., & Hung, L. O. (2004). Empowerment of patients with end-stage renal disease: A randomized controlled trial. *International Journal of Nursing Studies, 41*(1), 59–65.

Introduction

Tsay and Hung (2004) conducted a randomized controlled trial examining the effectiveness of an empowerment program on empowerment level, self-care self-efficacy, and depression in patients with end-stage renal disease (ESRD). The researchers used the Empowerment Scale, the Strategies Used by People to Promote Health Tool, and the Beck Depression Inventory to collect data from the patients on their level of empowerment, self-care self-efficacy, and depression, respectively. The scales were administered to both the control (*n* = 25) and the experimental (*n* = 25) groups at baseline and 6 weeks after the program was completed. The control group, experimental group, and total sample's empowerment, self-care self-efficacy, and depression baseline and posttest means and standard deviations are presented in Table 2 on p. 118.

Relevant Study Results

"The sample consisted of 50 hemodialysis patients. . . . Mean perceived renal disease severity was moderately severe (mean = 6.74, *SD* = 2.97, range = 0–10), and the mean length of dialysis was 52.56 months (*SD* = 36.51). There were no differences in clinical and demographic characteristics of the patients between the groups (*p* <0.05). The data indicates homogeneity of subjects across the groups" (Tsay & Hung, 2004, p. 61). "This study found that there were significant differences in improvement of empowerment, self-care self-efficacy, and depression in patients who were in the intervention group using empowerment strategies than with the control group patients.

. . .The results from this study suggest that empowerment techniques might have an important role for patients in self-management of ESRD. . . . The study provides a foundation for future studies of empowerment interventions for self-managing of ESRD patients" (Tsay & Hung, 2004, pp. 63–4).

TABLE 2 ■ Description of Studied Variables in Baseline and Post-test Between Groups						
	EXPERIMENT (*n* = 25)		CONTROL (*n* = 25)		TOTAL (*n* = 25)	
Variables	Mean	*SD*	Mean	*SD*	Mean	*SD*
Empowerment						
Baseline	98.40	9.19	97.08	8.99	97.74	9.02
Post-test	105.04	7.28	97.12	8.73	101.08	8.91
Self-care self-efficacy						
Baseline	89.56	14.88	93.00	13.62	91.28	14.02
Post-test	96.00	13.55	91.40	10.55	93.70	12.24
Depression						
Baseline	14.00	11.31	10.40	10.34	12.20	10.88
Post-test	13.36	10.55	10.40	10.34	11.88	10.45

Tsay, S. L., & Hung, L. O. (2004). Empowerment of patients with end-stage renal disease: A randomized controlled trial. *International Journal of nursing Studies, 41*(1), p. 62.

■ STUDY QUESTIONS

1. The research hypothesis for the Tsay and Hung (2004) study can be formulated as follows: "Patients with ESRD who obtain the empowerment program have higher levels of empowerment and self-care self-efficacy and are less depressed than those who do not receive the program." State the null hypothesis for this study.

2. What was the average baseline depression score of the experimental group subjects?

3. Compare the baseline and the posttest means of the self-care self-efficacy variable for the experimental group. Was this an expected finding? Provide a rationale for your answer.

4. Which group showed more variability or greater dispersion in their depression posttest scores? Provide a rationale for your answer.

5. What was the arithmetic average of all empowerment posttest scores collected in this study?

6. What variable was affected the most by the empowerment program? Is this an expected result? Provide a rationale for your answer.

7. On average, how long had the ESRD patients been on dialysis? Was there a significant difference between the control and the experimental groups in the length of time they had been on dialysis?

8. The self-care self-efficacy posttest's $\overline{X} = 96.00$ means that:
   a. the total sample for the study was 96 subjects.
   b. 96 was the average self-care self-efficacy posttest score for the experimental group.
   c. 96 was the lowest score the participants could get in order to be accepted into the experimental group.
   d. the difference between the experimental and control groups was 96 for self-efficacy.

9. The control group's baseline empowerment $SD = 8.99$. What does this statement mean?

ANSWERS TO STUDY QUESTIONS

1. The null hypothesis is: "There is no difference in the levels of empowerment, self-care self-efficacy, and depression of patients with ESRD who attend an empowerment program versus those who do not."

2. The average or mean baseline depression score of the experimental group was 14.00.

3. The experimental group's mean self-care self-efficacy posttest score (mean = 96.00) was 6.44 points higher than its baseline mean score (mean = 89.56) because on average the experimental group subjects scored higher on the posttest than at baseline or the beginning of the study. This was an expected finding because it was hypothesized that after the completion of the empowerment program, the experimental group's self-care self-efficacy skills would improve. This finding indicates that the empowerment intervention had a positive impact on the self-care self-efficacy of ESRD patients.

4. The experimental group's posttest scores were slightly more dispersed as demonstrated by the larger $SD = 10.55$, as opposed to the $SD = 10.34$ for the control group. But there is really minimal difference in the SD for both groups.

5. Mean = 101.08. The arithmetic average or mean of all empowerment posttest scores collected in this study was listed in Table 2 under total group mean.

6. The experimental subjects' mean empowerment scores showed the greatest increase from baseline to posttest, with a 6.64 point increase as compared to a 6.44 point increase for self-care self-efficacy and a 0.64 point decrease for depression. This is an expected result because the intervention was an empowerment program and one would expect that this type of program would have a greater effect on empowerment level and also on the self-care self-efficacy more than on the depression scores.

7. The Relevant Study Results indicated that the mean or average length of time on dialysis was 52.56 months. The article indicated that there was no significant difference between the control and experimental groups in clinical and demographic characteristics ($p <0.05$), so there was no significant difference in length on time on dialysis for the two groups.

8. Answer: b.   96 was the average self-care self-efficacy posttest score for the experimental group. Mean is an arithmetic average of the scores of a distribution (in this case, a distribution of the posttest self-care self-efficacy scores of the experimental group).

9. The control group's baseline empowerment $SD = 8.99$ indicates that one standard deviation from the mean for the empowerment variable equaled 8.99 and that this SD indicates the amount of dispersion or spread of the scores in the control group at baseline.

■ EXERCISE 16   Questions to be Graded

1. The researchers analyzed the data they collected as though it were at what level of measurement?
   a. Nominal
   b. Ordinal
   c. Interval/ratio
   d. Experimental

2. What was the mean posttest empowerment score for the control group?

3. Compare the mean baseline and posttest depression scores of the experimental group. Was this an expected finding? Provide a rationale for your answer.

4. Compare the mean baseline and posttest depression scores of the control group. Do these scores strengthen or weaken the validity of the research results? Provide a rationale for your answer.

5. Which group's test scores had the least amount of variability or dispersion? Provide a rationale for your answer.

6. Did the empowerment variable or self-care self-efficacy variable demonstrate the greatest amount of dispersion? Provide a rationale for your answer.

7. The mean $(\overline{X})$ is a measure of _____ _____ of a distribution while the SD is a measure of _____ of its scores. Both $\overline{X}$ and SD are _____ statistics.

8. What was the mean severity for renal disease for the research subjects? What was the dispersion or variability of the renal disease severity scores? Did the severity scores vary significantly between the control and the experimental groups? Is this important? Provide a rationale for your answer.

9. Which variable was least affected by the empowerment program? Provide a rationale for your answer.

10. Was it important for the researchers to include the total means and SDs for the study variables in Table 2 to promote the readers' understanding of the study results? Provide a rationale for your answer.

MEAN, STANDARD DEVIATION, AND 68% OF THE NORMAL CURVE

STATISTICAL TECHNIQUE IN REVIEW

The **mean** ($\bar{X}$) is a measure of central tendency and is the sum of the raw scores divided by the number of scores being summed. The **standard deviation** (*SD*) is calculated to determine the dispersion or spread of the scores from the mean. The larger the standard deviation value, the greater the variability of the scores from the mean. (See Exercise 16 for detailed information on mean and standard deviation.)

The theoretical normal curve is symmetrical and unimodal; thus, the mean, median, and mode are equal (see Figure 17-1). In a normal curve, 68% of the scores will be within one *SD* above or below the mean. Thus, 34% of the scores in a distribution lie above the mean and 34% below the mean (Burns & Grove, 2007). For example, if the $\bar{X} = 100$ and $SD = 20$, then 68% of the cases lie between 80 and 120, or within 20 points above and below the mean. The formula used to calculate the 68% rule to determine where 68% of the scores for the normal curve lie is:

Formula for Calculation of the 68% Rule is: $\bar{X} \pm SD$.

FIGURE 17-1 ■ Distribution of the Normal Curve and 68% of the Scores

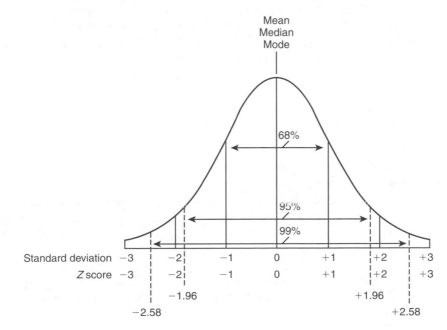

The data described below are the verbal scores for the individuals taking the graduate record exam (GRE) for one year with $\bar{X} = 490.0$ and $SD = 100$ (see Figure 17-2). Using the formula:

$$\bar{X} \pm SD = 490.0 \pm 100 = 490.0 + 100 = 590.0 \text{ and } 490.0 - 100 = 390.0$$

Thus, 68% of the scores in this distribution lie between the values of 390.0 and 590.0 and are expressed as (390.0, 590.0). Since 68% of the scores are between 390.0 and 590.0, this leaves 32% of the scores outside this interval. Since a normal curve is symmetric, one-half of the scores outside the interval, or 16%, are on each end of the distribution (see Figure 17-2).

FIGURE 17.2 ■ Distribution of GRE Scores on the Normal Curve.

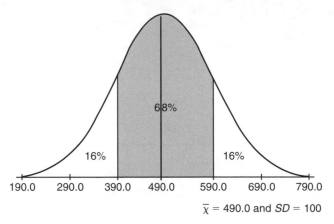

$\bar{\chi} = 490.0$ and $SD = 100$

RESEARCH ARTICLE

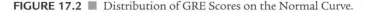

Source: Sjögren, T., Nissinen, K. J., Järvenpää, S. K., Ojanen, M. T., Vanharanta, H., & Mälkiä, E. A. (2005). Effects of workplace physical exercise intervention on the intensity of headache and neck and shoulder symptoms and upper extremity muscular strength of office workers: A cluster randomized controlled cross-over trial. *Pain, 116*(1–2), 119–28.

Introduction

Sjögren et al. (2005) examined the effects of physical exercise on intensity of headache and neck and shoulder pain. This randomized controlled trial consisted of 53 office workers who reported headache symptoms ($n = 41$) and/or pain in the neck ($n = 37$) or shoulders ($n = 41$) that restricted their activities of daily living during the last 12 months. "Physical exercise intervention resulted in a slight, but statistically significant, decrease in the intensity of headache and neck symptoms, as well as an increase in the extension strength of the upper extremities. . . . The intervention had no effect on intensity of shoulder symptoms or the flexion strength of the upper extremities. Specific exercise may be clinically important to alleviate headache and neck symptoms" (Sjögren et al., 2005, p. 119).

Relevant Study Results

"The purpose of this study was to examine the effects of a workplace physical exercise intervention, which consisted of light resistance training and guidance, on the perceived intensity of headache (i), the intensity of neck (ii) and shoulders symptoms (iii), as well as the muscular strength of the upper extremites (iv)" (Sjögren et al., 2005, p. 120). "Of the 90 volunteers, 53 met one or more of the inclusion criteria. These 53 subjects (43 women, 10 men, mean age 46.6 (8.4) years) were labeled the Pain Symptoms Group and were categorized into three partially overlapping Pain Symptoms Sub-groups: the Headache Symptoms Group (n=41; 33 women, 8 men), the Neck Symptoms groups (n=37; 30 women, 7 men), and the Shoulder Symptoms Group (n=41; 34 women, 7 men) . . . . Thirty-seven of the 90 volunteers, who did not meet any of the inclusion criteria, formed the Symptom-Free Group" (Sjögren et al., 2005, p. 122). Subjects were randomized into one of two groups, Treatment group 1 or Treatment group 2. Treatment group 1, n=36, received the physical exercise intervention for 15 weeks, and then received no intervention for 15 weeks. Treatment group 2, n=17, received no intervention for the first 15 weeks, and then received the physical exercise intervention for 15 weeks. "The individual level baseline information of the Pain Symptoms Group, and the intensity of the pain symptoms of the Pain Symptoms Sub-groups are presented in Table 1" (Sjögren et al., 2005, p. 122).

TABLE 1 ■ The Individual Level Baseline Information of the Pain Symptoms Group, and the Intensity of the Pain Symptoms of the Pain Symptoms Sub-Groups

	MEAN (SD)			
	All	Women	Men	P
	Mean *(SD)*			
1. Pain Symptoms Group (n = 53, 43 women, 10 men)				
Age, years	46.6 (8.4)	46.5 (8.7)	47.1 (7.2)	0.831
High (cm)	167.3 (8.3)	164.9 (6.2)	177.6 (7.6)	0.000
Weight (kg)	72.3 (15.4)	68.9 (13.0)	86.9 (16.9)	0.000
Upper extremity muscular strength, 1RM				
Flexion (kg)	50.2 (13.5)	44.3 (6.0)	73.4 (8.3)	0.000
Extension (kg)	38.0 (15.3)	31.6 (6.5)	62.6 (14.8)	0.000
2. Pain symptoms sub-groups	Mean *(SD)*			
Headache Symptoms Group (n = 41, 33 women, 8 men)				
Intensity of headache[a]	2.3 (2.5)	2.3 (2.4)	2.1 (2.9)	0.859
Neck Symptoms Group (n = 37, 30 women, 7 men)				
Intensity of neck symptoms[a]	2.4 (2.2)	2.2 (2.3)	3.1 (1.7)	0.308
Shoulder Symptoms Group (n = 41, 34 women, 7 men)				
Intensity of shoulder symptoms[a]	2.7 (2.6)	2.8 (2.6)	2.3 (2.9)	0.494

[a] Borg CR10 scale: 0–10.
Sjögren, T., Nissinen, K. J., Järvenpää, S. K., Ojanen, M. T., Vanharanta, H., & Mälkiä, E. A. (2005). Effects of workplace physical exercise intervention on the intensity of headache and neck and shoulder symptoms and upper extremity muscular strength of office workers: A cluster randomized controlled cross-over trial. *Pain 116*(1–2), p. 122. Permission granted by the International Association for the Study of Pain.

"The physical exercise intervention, resistance training and guidance together significantly decreased the intensity of headache ($p = 0.001$) in the Headache Symptoms Group and the intensity of neck symptoms ($p = 0.002$) in the Neck Symptoms Group. In the shoulder area, no significant effect of physical exercise intervention or light resistance training was found" (Sjögren et al., 2005, p. 124).

■ STUDY QUESTIONS

1. What was the mean age of the original 90 participants in this study?

2. What is the mean and standard deviation for weight of the women in this study for the Pain Symptoms Group?

3. Did the men or women have greater variability in their weight? Provide a rationale for your answer.

4. Assuming that the distribution of the women's weight is normal, 68% of the women's weights lie between what two values? Discuss what this result indicates.

5. Assuming that the distribution of age is normal for the study, what percentages of the original 90 volunteers were between 37.2 and 54.2 years of age? Show your calculations.

6. Assuming that the distribution for height is normal, what value represents one *SD* above the mean for the women's heights?

7. Assuming that the distribution of weight is normal for the study, what is the men's weight that is one *SD* below the mean? Show your calculations. What does this result indicate?

8. Assuming that the distribution of weight is normal for the sample of the Pain Symptoms Group, what would be the range of weight for 68% of subjects around the mean? Show your calculations.

9. Was the physical exercise intervention with resistance training and guidance effective in relieving intensity of neck symptoms? Provide a rationale for your answer.

■ ANSWERS TO STUDY QUESTIONS

1. The mean age was 45.7 years, which can be found in the Relevant Study Results from the research article.
2. The mean weight of women is 68.9 kg and $SD = 13.0$.
3. Men had greater variability in their weight with $SD = 16.9$ compared to women with $SD = 13.0$. The larger the value of standard deviation, the greater the variability or spread of the scores in a distribution.
4. The middle 68% of women's weights were between (55.9, 81.9)

    Calculation: $\bar{X} \pm SD$ $\bar{X} = 68.9$ $SD = 13.0$ $68.9 - 13.0 = 55.9$ kg $68.9 + 13.0 = 81.9$ kg

    The answer is expressed as (55.9, 81.9) and indicates that 68% of the women's weights are between a low of 55.9 kg and a high of 81.9 kg. This result indicates the spread or dispersion of the women's weights one SD above and below the mean for this study sample.
5. 68% of participants ages were between (37.2, 54.2) years with the $SD = 8.5$, $\bar{X} = 45.7$ years of age.

    Calculation: $\bar{X} \pm SD$ $45.7 + 8.5 = 54.2$ years of age $45.7 - 8.5 = 37.2$ years of age
6. Assuming that the distribution is normal, one SD above the mean for women's height in the Symptoms Group is 171.1 cm.

    Calculation: $\bar{X} + SD$ $\bar{X} = 164.9$ cm $SD = 6.2$ $164.9 + 6.2 = 171.1$ cm
7. Assuming that the distribution is normal, the men's weight one SD below the mean is 70 kg.

    Calculation: $\bar{X} \pm SD$ $\bar{X} = 86.9$ kg $SD = 16.9$ $86.9 - 16.9 = 70$ kg

    This result indicates that men with a weight one SD below the mean would weigh 70 kg.
8. Assuming that the distribution of weight is normal for the Pain Symptoms Group, 68% of the subjects would have a weight between 87.7 kg and 56.9 kg expressed as (56.9, 87.7).

    Calculation: $\bar{X} \pm SD$ $72.3 + 15.4 = 87.7$ kg $72.3 - 15.4 = 56.9$ kg
9. In combination with resistance training and guidance, the physical exercise intervention was effective in significantly decreasing the intensity of the neck symptoms as indicated by the $p = 0.002$. Any $p \leq 0.05$ indicates a statistically significant difference between the treatment and the comparison groups. Thus, the physical exercise treatment was effective in reducing the intensity of neck symptoms.

■ EXERCISE 17　Questions to be Graded

1. Assuming that the distribution for intensity of headache symptoms is normal, what percentage of women had headache intensity between 2.3 and 4.7?

2. Assuming that the scores are normally distributed, 68% of the subjects had scores between 0.1 and 5.3 for intensity of shoulder symptoms. Is this statement true or false? Provide a rationale for your answer.

3. Assuming that the distribution for upper extremity muscle flexion is normal, 68% of the subjects scored between what two values for upper extremity muscle flexion?

4. Assuming that the distribution for age is normal, what percentage of the Pain Symptom Group fell between the ages of 46.6 and 55 years? Provide a rationale for your answer.

5. For intensity of shoulder symptoms, did men or women have more variability in their scores? Provide a rationale for your answer.

6. A total of 34% of the men, one *SD* above the mean, had intensity of neck symptoms between 1.4 and 4.8. Is this statement true or false? Provide a rationale for your answer.

7. Assuming that the distribution for intensity of headache symptoms is normal, 68% of the female subjects' scores around the mean lie between what values? Show your calculations.

8. What are the values for one *SD* above and below the mean for the age of the male subjects in the Pain Symptoms Group?

9. Assuming that the distribution for upper extremity muscle strength extension is normal, which group had more variability of scores, men or women? Provide a rationale for the variability that you noted in the two groups.

10. The physical exercise intervention, resistance training and guidance together, significantly decreased the intensity of headache ($p = 0.001$) in the Headache Symptoms Group and the intensity of neck symptoms ($p = 0.002$) in the Neck Symptoms Group. What do these p values mean? What do these results indicate?

18

MEAN, STANDARD DEVIATION, AND 95% AND 99% OF THE NORMAL CURVE

STATISTICAL TECHNIQUE IN REVIEW

Mean ($\bar{X}$) is a measure of central tendency and is the sum of the raw scores divided by the number of scores being summed. **Standard deviation** (**SD**) is calculated to measure dispersion or the spread of scores from the mean (Burns & Grove, 2007). The larger the value of the standard deviation for study variables, the greater the dispersion or variability of the scores for the variable in a distribution. (See Exercise 16 for a detailed discussion of mean and standard deviation.)

Since the theoretical normal curve is symmetrical and unimodal, the mean, median, and mode are equal in the normal curve (see Figure 18-1). In the normal curve, 95% of the scores will be within 1.96 standard deviations of the mean, and 99% of scores are within 2.58 standard deviations of the mean. Figure 18-1 demonstrates the normal curve, with a $\bar{X} = 0$. The formula used to calculate the 95% rule to determine where 95% of the scores for the normal curve lie is:

$$\bar{X} \pm 1.96 \ (SD)$$

The formula used to calculate the 99% rule to determine where 99% of the scores for the normal curve lie is:

$$\bar{X} \pm 2.58 \ (SD)$$

FIGURE 18-1 ■ The Normal Curve

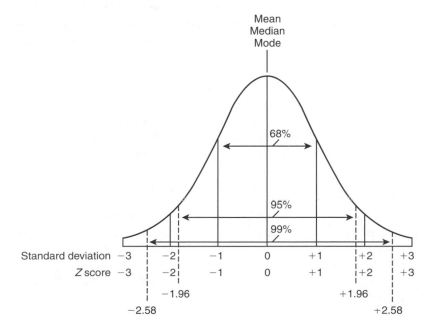

The data described below are the verbal SAT scores for high school seniors for one year with $\bar{X} = 490$ and $SD = 100$ (see Figure 18-2). The formula used to find where 95% of the scores lie is $\bar{X} \pm 1.96 \, (SD)$. In this example, $490 + 1.96 \, (100) = 686$, and $490 - 1.96 \, (100) = 294$. Thus 95% of scores lie between 294 and 686, expressed as (294, 686). Since 95% of the scores are between 294 and 686, this leaves 5% of the scores outside this interval. Since a normal curve is symmetric, one-half of the scores, or 2.5%, are at each end of this distribution.

To find where 99% of scores lie, $\bar{X} \pm 2.58 \, (SD)$, where $490 + 2.58 \, (100) = 748$ and $490 - 2.58 \, (100) = 232$. Thus, 99% of the SAT scores lie between 232 and 748, which is expressed as (232, 748). Since the distribution of these scores is normal, 99% of the scores are between 232 and 748 and 0.5% of the scores are at each end of this distribution.

FIGURE 18-2 ■ Distribution of SAT Scores

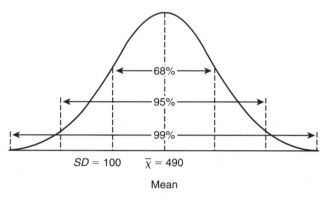

RESEARCH ARTICLE

Source: Corless, I. B., Nicholas, P. K., McGibbon, C. A., & Wilson, C., (2004). Weight change, body image, and quality of life in HIV disease: A pilot study. *Applied Nursing Research 17*(4), 292–6.

Introduction

The purpose of this pilot study [conducted by Corless and colleagues (2004)] was to investigate the relationships of weight change, body image, length of time with HIV/AIDS diagnosis, and quality of life in individuals with HIV disease (Corless et al., 2004, p. 292). The sample consisted of 40 subjects: 23 men and 17 women. The HIV-positive adults in a primary care clinic were asked to participate, so this study has a sample of convenience. The participants reported an increase in weight, greater than their ideal weight. The body image scores were found to be significantly higher for women, with the HIV-positive participants having slightly higher body image scores. A survey and Medical Outcomes Study–HIV (MOS-HIV) instruments were used as measurement methods for this study. The results indicated that when a person's weight is higher and closer to his or her ideal, HIV-positive individuals exhibit better quality of life. Thus, "education of clinicians and individuals living with HIV/AIDS should focus on the assessment, management, and evaluation of weight change during the course of HIV disease" (Corless et al., 2004, p. 292).

Relevant Study Results

"The sample consisted of 23 men with a mean age of 42.2 years ($SD = 8.2$), length of time since diagnosis with HIV was 9.2 years ($SD = 5.3$); and 17 women with a mean age of 36.8 years ($SD = 5.2$), and length of time since diagnosis with HIV was 7.2 years ($SD = 4.8$). For men, 23 were HIV-positive and 9 had a diagnosis of AIDS; and for women, 17 were HIV positive, and 5 had a diagnosis of AIDS. There was no significant difference in demographic characteristics of the sample by age, gender, HIV disease status, and time living with HIV.

Participants reported a net increase in weight from 3 months prior ($M = 2.4$ lb, $SD = 12.9$ lb) and 12 months prior ($M = 10.9$ lb, $SD = 19.1$ lb) and that their weight was greater than their ideal weight ($M = 9.2$ lb, $SD = 22.9$ lb). SDs for the data indicated a wide range on weight at both 3 and 12 months before participation in the study.

Body image scores (0–100 scale) were significantly ($F_{(1, 37)} = 5.41$, $p = .03$) higher for women (73.1 ± 17.0) than men (60.2 ± 17.0). Although HIV-positive participants had slightly higher body image scores ($M = 68.0$, $SD = 17.0$) compared with participants with AIDS ($M = 60.5$, $SD = 18.8$), there was no significant difference ($F_{(1, 37)} = 1.56$, $p = .22$) in body image scores between [those with HIV and AIDS]. There was a weak, but significant, inverse association between body image score and weight changes from 3 months prior ($r = -.30$, $p = .04$). Body image and weight scores are summarized in Table 1" (Corless et al., 2004, p. 294).

TABLE 1 ■ Body Image and Weight Measures for Men and Women

| | GENDER | | | |
| | Male | | Female | |
	Mean	SD	Mean	SD
Body image	60.22	16.98	73.07	16.93
Weight change last 12 months	10.26	22.40	11.94	13.63
Weight change last 3 months	3.05	15.87	1.47	7.32
Weight relative to ideal	5.48	22.93	14.44	22.57
Body weight ratio	53.66	33.97	67.56	34.44

Corless, I. B., Nicholas, P. K., McGibbon, C. A., & Wilson, C., (2004). Weight change, body image, and quality of life in HIV disease: A pilot study. *Applied Nursing Research, 17*(4), p. 294.

"A summary of quality-of-life scores for men and women is shown in Table 2. The scales of the MOS-HIV Quality of Life instrument include General Health Perceptions, Physical Functioning, Role Functioning, Social Functioning, Cognitive Functioning, Pain, Mental Health, Vitality, Health Distress, Quality of Life, and Heath Transition. There were no significant differences between quality of life scores between men and women. Men did have lower scores on some MOS-HIV scales (Cognitive Functioning, Pain, Quality of Life, and Health Transition) and women were lower on others (Vitality and Health Distress). In addition, there were a number of differences in the relationships between quality of life scores, body image, and body weight. . . . The positive correlations indicated that improved quality of life was associated with improved body image" (Corless et al., 2004, pp. 294–5).

TABLE 2 ■ Mean MOS-HIV Scores for Men and Women

| | GENDER | | | |
| | Male | | Female | |
	Mean	SD	Mean	SD
General health perceptions	37.38	30.52	39.71	25.46
Physical functioning	64.13	25.55	65.20	29.79
Role functioning	50.00	46.29	50.00	46.77
Social functioning	65.45	29.72	64.71	26.95
Cognitive functioning	58.86	30.94	66.18	26.55
Pain	52.53	30.90	64.71	28.12
Mental health	57.09	23.72	61.50	22.81
Vitality	48.86	23.35	43.24	21.93
Health distress	58.48	30.80	51.18	24.53
Quality of life	53.26	26.44	61.76	21.86
Health transition	56.52	24.09	66.18	24.91
Total MOS-HIV score	56.89	20.44	58.06	17.56

Corless, I. B., Nicholas, P. K., McGibbon, C. A., & Wilson, C., (2004). Weight change, body image, and quality of life in HIV disease: A pilot study. *Applied Nursing Research, 17*(4), p. 295.

■ STUDY QUESTIONS

1. In comparing men and women, which group had higher body image scores? Provide a rationale for your answer.

2. Men had higher variability in weight change over the last 12 months when compared to women. Is this statement true or false? Provide a rationale for your answer.

3. What are the $\bar{X}$ and SD values for men's body weight ratio?

4. Assuming that the distribution of scores is normal, calculate the scores where 95% of values around the mean lie for women with weight change over the last 3 months. Round your answer to two decimal places.

5. Assuming that the distribution of body weight ratio is a normal curve, 95% of the men lie between which two values of body weight ratio around the mean? Round your answer to two decimal places.

6. Assuming that the distribution of womens's body image scores is normal, 99% of women's body image scores around the mean lie between what two values? Round your answer to two decimal places.

7. Assuming that the distribution is a normal curve, 99% of men were between what ages? Round your answer to two decimal places.

8. Assuming that the distribution is a normal curve, 95% of men were between what ages? Round your answer to two decimal places.

9. Did HIV-positive participants have significantly higher body image scores than those with AIDS? Provide a rationale for your response.

■ ANSWERS TO STUDY QUESTIONS

1. Women had higher body image scores with a $\bar{X} = 73.07$ compared to men with a $\bar{X} = 60.22$. In this study, the greater the mean, the higher the body image scores. Thus, the higher mean for women's body image scores indicates that women have stronger body image scores than men.

2. True. *SD* indicates variability or spread of scores. Men had higher variability in scores with a $SD = 22.40$ versus women with a $SD = 13.63$. These results indicate that women had less variability in their weight over 12 months than men did in this study. Men often are more variable in their weight loss and gain, which is supported by this study.

3. $\bar{X} = 53.66$, $SD = 33.97$. These values are found in Table 1.

4. Assuming that the distribution of scores is normal, 95% of women's weight changes in the last 3 months were between (–12.88, 15.82).

$$\text{Calculation: } \bar{X} \pm 1.96(SD) \quad \bar{X} = 1.47 \quad SD = 7.32$$

$$1.47 - 1.96\,(7.32) = -12.877 = -12.88$$

$$1.47 + 1.96\,(7.32) = 15.817 = 15.82$$

$$\text{Expressed as } (-12.88, 15.82)$$

5. Assuming that the distribution of scores is normal for this sample, 95% of the men's body weight ratio values lie between (–12.92, 120.24).

$$\text{Calculation: } \bar{X} \pm 1.96(SD) \quad \bar{X} = 53.66 \quad SD = 33.97$$

$$53.66 - 1.96(33.97) = 53.66 - 66.58 = -12.92 \quad 53.66 + 1.96(33.97) = 53.66 + 66.58 = 120.24$$

$$\text{Expressed as } (-12.92, 120.24)$$

6. Assuming that the distribution of female body image scores is normal, 99% of the women's scores fall between (29.39, 116.75).

$$\text{Calculation: } \bar{X} \pm 2.58(SD) \quad \bar{X} = 73.07 \quad SD = 16.93$$

$$73.07 - 2.58(16.93) = 73.07 - 43.68 = 29.39 \quad 73.07 + 2.58\,(16.93) = 73.07 + 43.68 = 116.75$$

$$\text{Expressed as } (29.39, 116.75)$$

7. Assuming that the distribution of men's ages in the sample is normal, 99% of the men were between the ages (21.04, 63.36).

$$\text{Calculation: } \bar{X} \pm 2.58\,(SD) \quad \bar{X} = 42.2 \quad SD = 8.2$$

$$42.2 - 2.58(8.2) = 42.2 - 21.16 = 21.04 \quad 42.2 + 2.58(8.2) = 42.2 + 21.16 = 63.36$$

$$\text{Expressed as } (21.04, 63.36)$$

8. Assuming that the distribution of men's ages in the sample is normal, 95% of the men were between the ages (26.13, 58.27).

$$\text{Calculation: } \bar{X} \pm 1.96\,(SD) \quad \bar{X} = 42.2 \quad SD = 8.2$$

$$42.2 - 1.96(8.2) = 42.2 - 16.07 = 26.13 \quad 42.2 + 2.58(8.2) = 42.2 + 16.07 = 58.27$$

$$\text{Expressed as } (26.13, 58.27)$$

9. No. As found in the text of the Relevant Study Results, HIV-positive participants' mean score for body image was 68 compared to 60.5 for individuals with AIDS. These two groups were different in body image scores but were not significantly different, as indicated by $p = 0.22$. The $\alpha = 0.05$ was set prior to the conduct of the study; and since $p > 0.05$, the two groups are not significantly different in body image scores.

■ EXERCISE 18   Questions to be Graded

1. Assuming that the distribution is normal for weight relative to the ideal and 99% of the male participants scored between (–53.68, 64.64), where did 95% of the values for weight relative to the ideal lie? Round your answer to two decimal places.

2. Which of the following values from Table 1 tells us about variability of the scores in a distribution?
   a. 60.22
   b. 11.94
   c. 22.57
   d. 53.66

3. Assuming that the distribution for General Health Perceptions is normal, 95% of the females' scores around the mean were between what values? Round your answer to two decimal places.

4. Assuming that the distribution of scores for Pain is normal, 95% of the men's scores around the mean were between what two values? Round your answer to two decimal places.

5. Were the body image scores significantly different for women versus men? Provide a rationale for your answer.

6. Assuming that the distribution of Mental Health scores for men is normal, where are 99% of the men's mental health scores around the mean in this distribution? Round your answer to two decimal places.

7. Assuming that the distribution of scores for Physical Functioning in women is normal, where are 99% of the women's scores around the mean in this distribution? Round your answer to two decimal places.

8. Assuming that the distribution of scores is normal, 99% of HIV-positive body image scores around the mean were between what two values? Round your answer to two decimal places.

9. Assuming that the distribution of scores for Role Functioning is normal, 99% of the men's scores around the mean were between what values? Round your answer to two decimal places.

10. What are some of the limitations of this study that decrease the potential for generalizing the findings to the target population?

19 DETERMINING SKEWNESS OF A DISTRIBUTION

STATISTICAL TECHNIQUE IN REVIEW

The normal curve has a symmetrical or equal distribution of scores around the mean with a small number of outliers in the two tails. **Skewness** of a curve results in an asymmetrical distribution of scores around the mean with a number of outliers in one of the tails. The values of scores of a skewed distribution gravitate towards either extreme of their range (see Figures 19-1 and 19-2).

The skewness can be described as either positive or negative and refers to the location of the outlier scores of the distribution. A distribution is positively skewed when the tail with the outliers is to the right and the majority of its scores are congregated on the left side of the curve (see Figure 19-1). On the other hand, the outlier scores of a negatively skewed distribution are situated towards the left of the curve, while the "hump" comprising the majority of scores of a negatively skewed distribution is to the right side of the curve (see Figure 19-2). The formula for skewness is:

$$\text{Skewness} = \frac{\sum (X - \overline{X})^3}{N(SD^3)}$$

Skewness is usually calculated during data analysis, and the importance of the skewness needs to be determined by both the researcher and the statistician. Skewness $\geq +1$ or ≥ -1 is fairly severe and could impact the outcomes from parametric analysis techniques. Since the skewness or severity of the deviation from symmetry compromises the validity of the parametric tests,

FIGURE 19-1 ■ Positively Skewed Curve

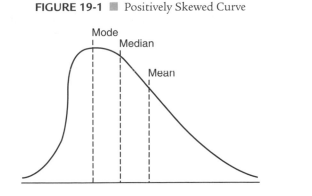

FIGURE 19-2 ■ Negatively Skewed Curve

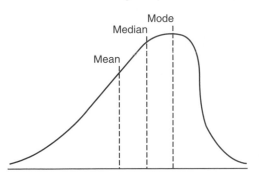

nonparametric analysis techniques are used to analyze the skewed interval or ratio level data. Nonparametric statistics have no assumption that the distribution of scores be normally distributed.

The mean, median, and mode of a skewed distribution are not equal to each other (see Figures 19-1 and 19-2); these values are equal only in the normally distributed curves. For example, in a positively skewed distribution, the numeric value of the mean will be greater than the value of the median, which will usually be greater than the value of the mode. In a negatively skewed distribution, the mode will be the largest value, followed by the median and then the mean (Burns & Grove 2005).

RESEARCH ARTICLE

Source: Björck Linné, A., Liedholm, S., Jendteg, S., & Israelsson, B. (2000). Health care costs of heart failure: Results from a randomized study of patient education. *European Journal of Heart Failure, 2*(3), 291–7.

Introduction

Björck Linné, Liedholm, Jendteg, and Israelsson (2000) described the health care costs of Swedish congestive heart failure (CHF) patients (*N* = 108) for a period of six months. The costs of hospitalization, outpatient visits, diagnostic tests and procedures, laboratory tests, and pharmacological therapy were analyzed separately to promote the readers' deeper understanding of the expenses associated with the condition. The results of the study revealed that the costs associated with the care of heart failure patients had a large inter-individual variation, formed a skewed distribution of values, and were the highest when hospitalization was needed.

Relevant Study Results

"The total cost (median) for a single heart failure patient was approximately 20,000 SEK (2,564 US$, 7.80 SEK = 1US$) for a 6-month period (Table 2)" (Björck Linné et al., 2000, p. 293).

TABLE 2 ■ Health Care Costs per Patient (in U.S. Dollars) during 6 Months of Follow-up after Hospitalization for Health Failure						
	Hospital Stay ($)	Out-Patient Visit ($)	Diagnostic Tests and Procedures	Laboratory Tests ($)	Drugs ($)	Total Costs ($)
Median	0	1,263	620	134	184	2,523
Range	0–11,568	0–5,000	14–8,279	0–515	8–427	590–16,025
Mean	1,761	1,398	900	148	173	4,380
SD	2,922	822	1,041	82	73	4,037

For comparison, data are displayed both as median and range and as mean and standard deviation.
The table was revised to show amounts in U.S. dollars from the original currency of Swedish Kronas at a rate of 7.80 Kronas to 1 U.S. Dollar. All values were rounded up to the nearest dollar.
Björck Linné, A., Liedholm, S., Jendteg, S., & Israelsson, B. (2000). Health care costs of heart failure: Results from a randomized study of patient education. *European Journal of Heart Failure, 2*(3), p. 293. Copyright © 2000, with permission from the European Society of Cardiology.

◼ STUDY QUESTIONS

1. The numeric value of the mode of a negatively skewed distribution is usually:
   a. smaller than the values of the mean and the median of that distribution.
   b. greater than the mean value of the distribution but smaller than its median value.
   c. greater than the median value of the distribution but smaller than its mean value.
   d. greater than the values of both the mean and the median of that distribution.

2. The age distribution of people diagnosed with heart failure is most likely to be:
   a. negatively skewed.
   b. normal.
   c. multimodal.
   d. positively skewed.

3. What measure of central tendency usually lies between the other two measures of central tendency regardless of the direction of the skewness of a distribution?
   a. Mean
   b. Median
   c. Mode
   d. Standard deviation

4. Determine the level of measurement of data collected by the researchers for this study. Provide a rationale for your answer.

5. In Table 2, median = 0 in the "Hospital stay" cost column. What is your interpretation of this study result?

6. In Table 1, the distribution of the hospitalization costs is:
   a. negatively skewed.
   b. normal distribution.
   c. not enough information provided to answer this question.
   d. positively skewed.

7. Describe the value of the mode of the distribution of the "Hospital stay" costs presented in Table 2.
   a. Mode equals zero.
   b. Since the researchers stated that there was a large inter-individual variation in costs, there was no mode.
   c. The mode is smaller than the mean, but there is really not enough information to calculate its exact value.
   d. The mode is greater than the mean.

8. Suppose that data from the participants who passed away during the study after a long period of hospitalization ($N=2$) were included in the study. How would these data change the distribution of the "Hospital stay" costs of CHF patients presented in Table 2?
   a. The distribution would be more positively skewed.
   b. The distribution of data of the hospital stay costs would form a normal curve.
   c. The distribution would be less positively skewed.
   d. The data would be skewed to the right or negatively skewed.

ANSWERS TO STUDY QUESTIONS

1. d.   Greater than the values of both the mean and the median of that distribution. The mode is the most frequently occurring score (the "hump" of a curve) and has a greater numerical value than the other measures of central tendency in a negatively skewed distribution. The median, which is unaffected by the outliers, is usually in the middle, reflecting the position of the 50th percentile. The mean, which is most sensitive to outlier influences (i.e., the lower scores of the distribution), is the smallest number in a negatively skewed distribution.

2. a.   Negatively skewed. Most heart failure patients are older individuals in their 60s to 90s, so the values of the age distribution of people with this condition are likely to gravitate towards the end of the human lifespan, or to the right of the curve. On the other hand, the "outliers" will be the younger individuals in the left tail of the curve.

3. b.   Median. In a positively skewed distribution, the mean is greater than the mode with the median situated in between the two values. In a negatively skewed distribution, the mean is the smallest number, mode is the largest, and the median is somewhere in between the mean and the mode. The standard deviation is not a measure of central tendency; it is a measure of dispersion.

4. Interval/ratio level data. Since researchers used the exact amounts of Swedish Kronas (SEK) to describe the costs associated with caring for patients with CHF, the data they collected was precise and had a continuum of values with equal distances between the intervals of the monetary values. Thus, money is considered a measurement at the interval/ratio level. The number of diagnostic tests and procedures are also interval/ratio data. No distinction is made between interval and ratio data since the analysis techniques are the same for both interval and ratio data (Burns & Grove, 2007).

5. The median hospital stay costs are $0, indicating at least 50% of the study participants had not been hospitalized during the duration of the study. Remember that the median is the score that lies in the middle of a rank ordered list of values of a distribution. Since the median cost for hospitalization of 108 patients equaled 0, no patients numbering 1 through 54 (50% of the sample) were hospitalized.

6. d.   Positively skewed. As explained in Question 5, most participants of the study were not hospitalized, so their hospitalization costs equaled $0. The outliers or CHF patients with the highest hospitalization costs are in the right tail of the curve resulting in a positively skewed distribution.

7. a.   Mode equals zero. Remember that the mode is the most frequently occurring score of a distribution, and the mode is less than the median in a positively skewed distribution (see Figure 19-1). Since the median is $0 hospitalization costs, then the mode, which is less than the median, is also $0 hospitalization costs.

8. c.   The distribution would be less positively skewed. There would be two more cases with longer hospitalizations that would slightly decrease the ratio of non-hospitalized to hospitalized patients, who were charged hospitalization fees. Thus, the degree of skewness of the curve would decrease and result in a less positively skewed curve.

■ EXERCISE 19   Questions to be Graded

1. The age distribution of people diagnosed with cystic fibrosis is most likely to be:
   a. negatively skewed.
   b. normally distributed.
   c. positively skewed.
   d. bimodal.

2. The numeric value of the mean of a positively skewed distribution is:
   a. smaller than both the median and the mode of that distribution.
   b. greater than the mode but smaller than the median of the distribution.
   c. greater than both the median and the mode.
   d. equal to both the median and the mode of the distribution.

3. Does a set of scores with most of its values above the mean have a negatively or positively skewed distribution? Provide a rationale for your answer.

4. Based on the results presented in Table 2, which of the therapeutic interventions did every participant receive during the study timeframe? Provide a rationale for your answer.

5. In Table 2, the distribution of the laboratory test costs is:
   a. positively skewed.
   b. negatively skewed.
   c. normal.
   d. not enough information provided to answer this question.

6. Based on the mean and median values of the cost categories presented in Table 2, which one of them has a negatively skewed distribution of values? Provide a rationale for your answer.

7. Based on the results presented in Table 2, which of the following statements is correct?
   a. Most patients chose to refuse medical services.
   b. Most patients had their condition under control during the study.
   c. Most patients of the study are in the late stages of heart failure.
   d. Most participants of the study had a severe and difficult to control condition.

8. Which of the cost distribution categories in Table 2 most closely resembles a normal curve?
   a. "Diagnostic tests and procedures"
   b. "Outpatient visits"
   c. "Drugs"
   d. "Total costs"

9. Why do you think the researchers included both the means and the medians in Table 2? What measure of central tendency would have described the sample most accurately? Provide a rationale for your answer.

10. Calculate the skewness of the following data set of pulse values for patients who have hypertension (HTN) and are being treated with beta blockers. Pulse values are: 65, 60, 60, 65, 80. The standard deviation (SD) = 8.22.

UNDERSTANDING *T* SCORES

STATISTICAL TECHNIQUE IN REVIEW

The **T score** is a type of standard score that is based upon the normal curve with a mean of 50 and a standard deviation of 10 for the norm group. Test developers have derived norm tables that allow us to convert a person's raw score (points earned) to the *T* score equivalents that would have been obtained if that person had been in the norm group. *T* scores permit a more meaningful comparison with a norm group than raw scores. Tests for admission to graduate and undergraduate schools (e.g., the Graduate Record Exam) typically use this type of standardized score. The formula frequently used for *T* score calculation is:

$$T \text{ score} = \frac{10X}{\text{SD}} + (50 - \frac{10\overline{X}}{SD})$$

Where: X = raw score to be converted
$\overline{X}$ = mean of the group of raw scores
SD = standard deviation of the raw scores

Example: Convert a raw score of 80 to a *T* score, where $\overline{X}$ = 75 and SD = 5.

$$T \text{ score} = \frac{10(80)}{5} + (50 - \frac{10(75)}{5}) = 160 + (50 - 150) = 160 - 100 = 60$$

RESEARCH ARTICLE

Source: LoGalbo, A., Sawrie, S., Roth, D. L., Kuzniecky, R., Knowlton, R., Faught, E., & Martin, R. (2005). Verbal memory outcome in patients with normal preoperative verbal memory and left mesial temporal sclerosis. *Epilepsy and Behavior, 6*(3), 337–41.

Introduction

LoGalbo et al. (2005) conducted a study to examine the "risk of verbal memory loss in patients with known structural abnormality (i.e., left mesial temporal sclerosis by MRI) and normal preoperative verbal memory performance who undergo left ATL [anterior temporal lobectomy]" (LoGalbo et al., 2005, p. 337). The researchers found that the "patients exhibiting normal presurgical verbal memory are at risk for verbal memory declines following ATL. These results suggest that functional integrity of the left mesial temporal lobe may play an important role in the verbal memory outcome in this patient group" (LoGalbo et al., 2005, p. 337). However, the researchers do recognize the limitations of their study and note that the small sample size restricts the generalization of the study findings.

Relevant Study Results

"Seventeen patients with left temporal epilepsy, MRI-based exclusive left MTS [mesial temporal sclerosis], and normal preoperative verbal memory were identified" (LoGalbo et al., 2005, p. 337). MTS is a structural abnormality in the brain. "The patients selected for the study were considered to have 'normal' preoperative verbal memory, defined as having preoperative performance across the learning (Acquisition) and long delayed free recall (Retrieval) portions of the California Verbal Learning Test (CVLT) of at least a *T* score above 40 (> 16%ile). The CVLT Acquisition score is the total number of words recalled across the five learning trials. The CVLT Retrieval score is defined as total number of words freely recalled after a 20-min delay. Both of these variables have been extensively employed as markers of verbal memory outcome following ATL [anterior temporal lobectomy] in several studies" (LoGalbo et al., 2005, p. 339). Clinical characteristics of these patients are summarized in Table 2, and average CVLT Acquisition and Retrieval *T* scores are presented in Table 3.

"The average drop in CVLT Acquisition *T* scores was 6.9, representing a decline of 15% from baseline performance. The average drop in CVLT Retrieval *T* scores was 9.6, representing a decline on average of 20% from baseline score" (LoGalbo et al., 2005, p. 340).

TABLE 2 ■ CVLT Acquisition and Retrieval *T* Scores for each Patient

Patient	Age	Gender	Education (years)	Age at Seizure Onset	WADA[a]		CVLT ACQUISITION[b]		CVLT RETRIEVAL[b]	
					L	R	Preop	Postop	Preop	Postop
1	34	F	13	17	8	6	44	48	51	47
2	53	M	12	4 Months	–	–	42	50	51	51
3	25	F	14	13	9	5	63	51	58	58
4	34	M	12	12	11	10	46	30	44	23
5	30	F	12	17	12	12	51	47	52	40
6	26	M	12	5	11	12	48	36	52	40
7	19	M	12	6	–	–	42	46	44	44
8	28	M	11	13	9	13	46	38	45	36
9	24	F	10	2	–	–	50	38	54	37
10	38	F	12	10	–	–	42	34	41	37
11	34	M	14	1	11	11	44	45	42	34
12	48	F	13	22	10	9	42	34	48	31
13	25	F	12	12	10	8	45	41	60	39
14	34	F	15	4	–	–	46	31	41	24
15	31	M	14	7	–	–	44	40	50	46
16	17	M	12	6	–	–	46	37	44	35
17	17	M	10	1	9	12	47	39	46	46

[a] L, left injection memory score (max value = 15); R, right injection memory score (max value = 15).
[b] California Verbal Learning Test (CVLT) scores are reported as *T* scores.

LoGalbo, A., Sawrie, S., Roth, D. L., Kuzniecky, R., Knowlton, R., Faught, E., & Martin, R. (2005). Verbal memory outcome in patients with normal preoperative verbal memory and left mesial temporal sclerosis. *Epilepsy and Behavior, 6*(3), p. 339. Copyright © 2005, with permission from Elsevier, Inc.

TABLE 3 ■ Average CVLT Acquisition and Retrieval *T* Scores and SRB Change Scores

	ACQUISITION	RETRIEVAL
Preoperative *T score*	45.9(5.2)	47.8(5.8)
Postoperative *T score*	39.0(7.2)	38.2(9.0)
SRB change scores	−1.0(.73)	−2.5(1.5)

LoGalbo, A., Sawrie, S., Roth, D. L., Kuzniecky, R., Knowlton, R., Faught, E., & Martin, R. (2005). Verbal memory outcome in patients with normal preoperative verbal memory and left mesial temporal sclerosis. *Epilepsy and Behavior, 6*(3), p. 340.

■ STUDY QUESTIONS

1. Which patients scored the lowest on the preoperative CVLT Acquisition? What was their *T* score?

2. Which patient scored the highest on postoperative CVLT Retrieval? What was this patient's *T* score?

3. Did the patient in Question 2 have a decline in memory retrieval performance from before and after surgery? Provide a rationale for your answer.

4. If a patient scored < 16%ile on the CVLT, what would his/her *T* score be less than?

5. What is the mean ($\bar{X}$) and standard deviation (*SD*) for preoperative *T* score for CVLT Retrieval?

6. Is the postoperative Acquisition *T* score for Patient 14 above or below the mean for the norm group? Provide a rationale for your answer.

7. Discuss the change in CVLT Acquisition *T* scores for Patient 14 from before and after surgery. How do her *T* scores compare with the mean CVLT Acquisition *T* scores before and after surgery? What do these results indicate about this patient's memory?

8. Assuming that the distribution of scores for the postoperative Acquisition is normal, the middle 68% of the patients had *T* scores between what two values?

9. If a patient had a raw score = 50, what would his/her preoperative CVLT Acquisition *T* score be?

ANSWERS TO STUDY QUESTIONS

1. Patients 2, 7, 10, and 12 have the lowest score on the preoperative CVLT Acquisition. The *T* score for all four patients was a 42 (see Table 2).

2. Patient 3 scored the highest on the postoperative CVLT Retrieval with a *T* score = 58 (see Table 2).

3. Patient 3 did not demonstrate a decline in memory retrieval performance from before and after surgery. This patient's *T* score was 58 preoperatively and postoperatively on the CVLT Retrieval, which means that the recall of words after a 20-minute delay was the same before and after surgery.

4. If a patient scored < 16%ile on the CVLT, his/her *T* score would be less than 40 as indicated in the Relevant Study Results from the article.

5. For preoperative Retrieval, the mean ($\bar{X}$) = 47.8 and the standard deviation (*SD*) = 5.8 (see Table 3).

6. Patient 14 had a postoperative Acquisition *T* score below the norm group mean, since her *T* score = 31 and the postoperative Acquisition norm group mean *T* score = 39.0.

7. Patient 14 had a preoperative Acquisition *T* score = 46, which was comparable to the mean preoperative CVLT Acquisition *T* score = 45.9. However, patient 14 had a postoperative Acquisition *T* score = 31, which was 8 points below the postoperative Acquisition norm group mean *T* score = 39. Patient 14 had a 15-point decline from before and after surgery when the average drop in the CVLT Acquisition *T* score was 6.9. Thus, this patient had a memory decline that was twice that of the other patients.

8. 68% of the scores for the postoperative CVLT Acquisition were between (31.8, 46.2)
Formula for 68% of the scores for a distribution is:

$$\bar{X} \pm SD \qquad \bar{X} = \mathbf{39.0} \qquad SD = \mathbf{7.2}$$

$$39.0 + 7.2 = 46.2 \qquad 39.0 - 7.2 = 31.8$$

9. $T \text{ score} = \dfrac{10X}{SD} + \left(50 - \dfrac{10X}{SD}\right)$

Raw score of *X* = 50 to a *T* score, where $\bar{X}$ = 45.9 and *SD* = 5.2.

$$T \text{ score} = \frac{10(50)}{5.2} + \left(50 - \frac{10(45.9)}{5.2}\right) = 96.15 + (50 - 88.27) = 96.15 - 38.27 = 57.88$$

■ EXERCISE 20   Questions to be Graded

1. Which patient scored the highest on the preoperative CVLT Acquisition? What was his or her T score?

2. Which patient scored the lowest on postoperative CVLT Retrieval? What was this patient's T score?

3. Did the patient in Question 2 have more of a memory performance decline than average on the CVLT Retrieval? Provide a rationale for your answer.

4. What is the mean ($\bar{X}$) and standard deviation (SD) for preoperative T score for CVLT Acquisition?

5. Is the preoperative Retrieval T score for Patient 5 above or below the mean for the norm of the group? Provide a rationale for your answer.

6. Assuming that the distribution of the preoperative CVLT Retrieval *T* scores is normal, the middle 68% of the patients had *T* scores between what two values?

7. Assuming that the distribution of scores for the postoperative CVLT Retrieval *T* scores is normal, the middle 68% of the patients had *T* scores between what two values?

8. The researchers state that it appears that the functional integrity of the left temporal lobe, despite evidence of structural abnormality, plays a considerable role when it comes to memory outcomes following left ATL. Can the findings from this study be generalized to a larger population? Provide a rationale for your answer.

9. If a patient had a raw score = 30, what would his/her postoperative CVLT Retrieval *T* score be?

10. Did patients demonstrate more postoperative memory declines among CVLT Retrieval *T* scores than CVLT Acquisition *T* scores? Provide a rationale for your answer.

EFFECT SIZE

STATISTICAL TECHNIQUE IN REVIEW

Effect is the presence of the phenomenon in the population under investigation. **Effect size** is the degree to which this phenomenon is present and is reported as a numerical value. If a study focused on the effect of an 1,800 calorie diet on weight loss in adults, the effect size could be calculated to determine the effectiveness of the treatment in promoting the outcome of weight loss. The effect size (*ES*) can be calculated by subtracting the mean of the control or comparison group from the mean of the experimental group and dividing the difference by the standard deviation (*SD*) of the control or comparison group. The formula is presented below:

$$ES = (\overline{X} \textbf{ experimental group} - \overline{X} \textbf{ control group}) \div SD \textbf{ control group}$$

According to Burns and Grove (2005), a small *ES* is < 0.3 or –0.3, a medium *ES* ranges between 0.3 and 0.5 or –0.3 and –0.5, and a large *ES* is > 0.5 or > –0.5. Please note that depending on the numeric values of the means of the control and experimental groups, the effect sizes can be positive or negative. Negative effect sizes indicate that the mean of the control group was larger than the mean of the experimental group, but the opposite is true for the positive effect sizes.

The effect size for a relationship is equal to the value calculated for the relationship. For example, the correlation of pulse and respiration can be calculated with Pearson Product Moment Correlation Coefficient with $r = 0.56$. The effect size for the pulse and respiration relationship equals r value, so in this study $ES = r = 0.56$.

Effect size is one of the most essential determinants of the sample size needed to conduct a particular study. Small effect sizes are difficult to detect, so they require large samples to detect them, while large effect sizes can be easily detected with small samples. In turn, the sample size contributes to the study's ability to detect the presence of the effect of the phenomenon under study, that is, to correctly reject the null hypothesis. Using the example above, the null hypothesis is: "Adults consuming an 1,800 calorie diet have no greater weight loss than those adults consuming a regular diet." The ability of a study to correctly reject the null hypothesis is called **power** while the adequacy of its sample size is examined by performing a **power analysis** (see Exercise 12). A study should have a minimal power of 0.8 to detect significant differences or relationships in the study. This means that the study has an 80% probability of accurately detecting the presence of the phenomenon being investigated (Burns & Grove, 2007).

RESEARCH ARTICLE

Source: Rakel, B., & Frantz, R. (2003). Effectiveness of transcutaneous electrical nerve stimulation on postoperative pain with movement. *The Journal of Pain, 4*(8), 455–64.

Introduction

Rakel and Frantz (2003) examined the effectiveness of transcutaneous electrical nerve stimulation (TENS) as an adjunct to pharmacologic analgesia on postoperative pain with movement after abdominal surgery. They also evaluated its impact on patients' pain, vital capacity maneuvers, and walking parameters, such as gait speed, gait distance, and the level of assistance required. Three pain control strategies were randomly assigned to each of the first 3 ambulations on a postoperative day: (1) pharmacologic analgesia and TENS, (2) pharmacologic analgesia and placebo TENS, and (3) pharmacologic analgesia alone. TENS electrodes were applied parallel to the incision on both sides, and the frequency was self-adjusted by patients to as high a level as they could tolerate. Patient frequency selections ranged between 3 and 57 mA. Based on the TENS frequency they used, the patients ($N = 33$) were divided into 2 groups: a high frequency group (≥ 9 mA) and a low frequency group (≤ 8 mA). Use of TENS resulted in significantly lower pain intensity ratings during walking and vital capacity maneuvers, and faster gait and greater gait distances than with using analgesia alone. The patients' pain with movement was measured with a vertical 21-item numeric rating scale (NRS) during transfer from lying to sitting position, walking, and performing vital capacity maneuvers. These data were analyzed with means and standard deviations, which are presented in Table 1.

Relevant Study Results

"A prospective, randomized, repeated measures design was used. Subjects served as their own controls. . . An estimation of desired sample size for dependent groups was determined by using pain intensity scores of the first 13 study subjects. On the basis of the effect sizes ranging between 0.22 for TENS versus placebo TENS and 0.77 for TENS versus pharmacologic analgesia alone, a moderate

TABLE 1 ■ Descriptive Statistics for Pain Intensity During Transfer, Gait Speed, Gait Distance, and Vital Capacity

		TENS INTENSITY					
		Mean	*SD*	*Mean*	*SD*	*Mean*	*SD*
	Treatment	High (≥ 9 mA)		Low (≤ 8 mA)		Total Sample	
Transfer		(n = 19)		(n = 13)		(N = 32)	
	TENS	9.5	5.898	10.5	4.539	9.9	5.330
	Placebo	11.1	5.641	11.2	5.031	11.1	5.318
	Control	10.7	4.711	10.8	4.560	10.7	4.576
Gait speed		(n = 16)		(n = 12)		(N = 28)	
	TENS	6.9	3.714	9.8	4.808	8.1*	4.369
	Placebo	9.1	4.299	11.1	4.641	9.9	4.483
	Control	10.2	4.175	9.8	3.129	10.1*	3.702
Gait distance		(n = 20)		(n = 13)		(N = 33)	
	TENS	9.3	3.932	9.6	4.930	9.4	4.280
	Placebo	9.5	4.691	10.2	4.902	9.8	4.712
	Control	11.1	3.967	10.8	3.018	11.0	3.576
Vital capacity		(n = 18)		(n = 12)		(N = 30)	
	TENS	7.8	4.579	7.9	4.448	7.8*†	4.450
	Placebo	9.7	5.594	9.9	4.776	9.8*	5.197
	Control	11.0	3.629	9.1	4.101	10.2†	3.876

Abbreviation: *SD*, standard deviation
* Significantly different at $p < .05$
† Significantly different at $p < .01$
Rakel, B. Frantz, R. (2003). Effectiveness of transcutaneous electrical nerve stimulation on postoperative pain with movement. *The Journal of Pain, 4*(8), p. 459. Copyright © 2003, with permission from The American Pain Society.

effect size was assumed. . . α = .05 and power = .7 required a sample size of 24 subjects" (Rakel & Frantz, 2003, p. 456). "The highest effect was between TENS and pharmacologic analgesia for pain during vital capacity (–0.58), followed by pain during gait speed (–0.47). The lowest effect sizes were between placebo TENS and pharmacologic analgesia alone for pain during gait speed (–0.03) and pain during transfer (0.08)" (p. 459).

■ STUDY QUESTIONS

1. Which group served as the control group in this study?
   a. The group that used placebo TENS
   b. The group that used analgesia alone
   c. The group that used TENS in addition to analgesia
   d. The group that tolerated using their TENS set at high frequency amplitude (≥ 9 mA)

2. Using data presented in Table 1, calculate the *ES* of the TENS for the total sample subjects' pain intensity during the gait distance maneuver. Show your calculations and round your answer to two decimal places. Was there a significant difference in pain intensity during the gait distance maneuver between the TENS and control groups?

3. Was the *ES* calculated in Question 2 small, medium, or large? Was it a positive or a negative value? Was it expected that the result would be positive/negative? Provide a rationale for your answer.

4. Using data presented in Table 1, calculate the *ES* of placebo TENS for the total sample subjects' pain intensity during the gait distance maneuver. Show your calculations and round your answer to two decimal places. Is the *ES* larger or smaller than the one obtained in Question 2? Was this expected? Provide a rationale for your response.

5. Using data presented in Table 1, calculate the *ES* of TENS for the total sample subjects' pain intensity during the vital capacity maneuver. Show your calculations and round your answer to two decimal places. Which maneuver was affected by using TENS in addition to analgesia to a greater degree, the gait distance or the vital capacity? Provide a rationale for your answer.

6. The larger the effect size, the larger the sample required to detect significant differences in a study. Is this statement true or false? Provide a rationale for your answer.

7. Based on the *ES* value calculated in Question 3, was the power of this study adequate to reject the null hypothesis? Provide a rationale for your answer.

8. An inadequate sample size can cause all of the following except:
   a. decrease the power of a study.
   b. result in a false acceptance of the null hypothesis.
   c. compromise the validity of the results.
   d. increase the effect size.

9. The power of this study could be increased by:
   a. increasing the size of the sample.
   b. decreasing the *ES*.
   c. adding more variables.
   d. adding another experimental group.

■ ANSWERS TO STUDY QUESTIONS

1. b.   The group that used analgesia alone. The purpose of the study was to evaluate the effectiveness of the TENS therapy as an adjunct to pharmacological analgesia, so the group that received the TENS plus analgesia was the experimental group and the group that received analgesia alone was the control group. The group that received the placebo TENS was manipulated by the researchers (a TENS unit was attached even though no treatment was administered) and was called the placebo group. The researchers were comparing the effectiveness of analgesic treatments alone to the placebo group who received analgesia combined with TENS that was not turned on.

2. $ES = -0.45$. $ES = (9.4 - 11.0) \div 3.576 = -1.6 \div 3.576 = -0.447 = -0.45$. According to Table 1, use of TENS in addition to analgesia did not result in a significant decrease in pain scores between the experimental and the control group subjects. Significant results in Table 1 are marked by an asterisk (*) for significant differences at $p < .05$ or the † symbol that indicates significant differences at $p < .01$.

3. $ES = -0.45$ is a medium, negative effect size. ES values between –0.3 and –0.5 are considered to be of medium strength (Burns & Grove, 2007). The result was a negative number because it was obtained by subtracting the mean pain intensity score of the control group (a larger number) from the mean pain intensity score of the experimental group (a smaller number). The researchers expected that the pain intensity scores of the experimental group (treated with both TENS and analgesia) would be lower that those of the control group treated with analgesia alone.

4. $ES = -0.34$. $ES = (9.8 - 11.0) \div 3.576 = -1.2 \div 3.576 = -0.336 = -0.34$. Placebo TENS had a smaller effect on the pain intensity scores of study subjects than did the real TENS therapy ($ES = -.45$). The researchers expected that the TENS would result in a greater degree of pain relief for the subjects of the experimental group than a placebo unit would. In fact, the researchers probably hoped that the ES calculated in this question would be even smaller than it was. Even though the placebo TENS affected the pain intensity of the research subjects to a lesser degree than the real TENS, its ES is still medium (–0.34), as was the ES of the TENS unit treatment (–0.45).

5. $ES = -0.62$. $ES = (7.8 - 10.2) \div 3.876 = -2.4 \div 3.876 = -0.619 = -0.62$. The treatment of TENS with pharmacological therapy resulted in a greater decrease in pain intensity during the vital capacity maneuver than during the gait distance maneuver. The $ES = -0.62$ for pain intensity during vital capacity maneuver was larger than the $ES = -0.45$ calculated for the pain intensity during gait distance maneuver in Question 2. The larger the ES calculated for a study, the greater the effect of the treatment on the dependent variables measured in this study.

6. False. Large effect size indicates that the treatment was very effective and that it is easier to detect significant differences between groups, even with small sample sizes. Small effect size requires a larger sample to detect differences between groups.

7. No, the study did not have adequate power, and a larger sample was needed to detect significant differences in this study. Even though the effect size of the TENS on the pain intensity scores of the experimental group was medium ($ES = -0.45$), significant results were not obtained for the gait distance maneuver. Thus, the null hypothesis was accepted for the gait distance maneuver in this study. With a larger sample, statistically significant results would have probably been obtained and the null hypothesis rejected.

8. d.   Increase the effect size. An inadequate sample size decreases the power of the study, can result in false acceptance of the null hypothesis, and compromises the validity of the study results but cannot increase the ES. The ES indicates the effectiveness of the treatment and increases when the treatment is more effective or a strong relationship exists between study variables, but not with an increase in sample size.

9. a.   Increasing the size of the sample. This would have increased the power of this study. Decreasing the ES, adding more variables, and adding another experimental group all decrease the power of a study and make it more difficult to detect significant differences.

■ EXERCISE 21   Questions to be Graded

1. Why did researchers choose to include a placebo TENS group in this study?

2. In Table 1, which movement maneuver was least painful for control subjects in the low amplitude group? Provide a rationale for your answer.

3. Using data presented in Table 1, calculate the *ES* of TENS for the total sample subjects' pain intensity during transfer. Show your calculations and round your answer to two decimal places. Was the result significant? Provide a rationale for your answer.

4. How would you characterize the *ES* calculated in Question 3?
   a. Small
   b. Medium
   c. Large
   d. Non-existent

5. Based on the description of the sample size determination procedure provided in the Relevant Study Results, what was the most likely reason for the absence of significant differences between the levels of pain intensity of the experimental and the control groups undergoing the transfer procedure? Provide a rationale for your answer.

6. Using data presented in Table 1, calculate the *ES* of TENS for the total sample subjects' pain intensity during the gait speed maneuver. Show your calculations and round your answer to two decimal places. Was the result significant? Provide a rationale for your answer.

7. Does the fact that the highest effect sizes were observed between TENS/pharmacologic analgesia and pharmacologic analgesia alone and the lowest effect sizes were between placebo TENS/pharmacologic analgesia and pharmacologic analgesia alone (see the Relevant Study Results) strengthen or weaken the validity of the research hypothesis of this study? Provide a rationale for your answer.

8. Why did researchers divide the TENS group into the low and high amplitude groups?
   a. To compare the effects of both low and high amplitude TENS on patients' pain intensity during different maneuvers.
   b. To prove that only TENS set at high amplitude should be used as an adjunct therapy to pharmacological analgesia.
   c. To show that the subjects of the high amplitude group did not need pharmacologic analgesia to control their pain.
   d. By taking a closer look at the study, it is evident that the high amplitude group served as an experimental group while the low amplitude group served as a control group in this study.

9. What does it mean to design a study with a power of 1? Is this possible? Provide a rationale for your answer.

10. Based on the description of the study design presented in the Relevant Study Results, what does "subjects served as their own controls" mean?

SCATTERPLOT

STATISTICAL TECHNIQUE IN REVIEW

Scatterplots or scattergrams are used to describe relationships and provide a graphic picture of data. Variables are illustrated on two axes, x and y. The x-axis is the horizontal axis, and the y-axis is the vertical axis. To provide a visual image of the data, each point on the graph is a subject's scores for variables x and y, thus representing the relationship between the x and y variables on the graph. Each subject's scores on the two variables are plotted on the graph, and the number of points on the graph depends on the study sample size. The display of points on the graph indicates the direction (positive or negative) and strength (weak, moderate, or strong) of the relationship. For example, plots moving from the upper left corner to the lower right corner indicate an inverse or negative relationship (see Figure 22-1). Scatterplots moving from the lower left corner to the upper right corner, on the other hand, indicate a direct or positive relationship (see Figure 22-2). The closer the plotted points are to each other and the more they form a straight line, the stronger the linear relationship (see Figures 22-1 and 22-2). Conversely, if the plotted points are further away from each other and spread wide across the graph, this indicates a weak relationship that is closer to 0 (see Figure 22-3). When looking at scatterplots, it is important to identify outliers. **Outliers** are extreme values in the data set, which occur with inherent variability, measurement error, execution error, and error in identifying the variables. Outliers skew the data set and are an exception to the overall findings of the study. Figure 22-3 has examples of two outliers in the upper right corner. Researchers use scatterplots to identify linear and nonlinear relationships, but the focus of this exercise is understanding linear relationships (Burns & Grove, 2005).

RESEARCH ARTICLE

Source: Hitchings, E., & Moynihan, P. J. (1998). The relationship between television food advertisements recalled and actual foods consumed by children. *Journal of Human Nutrition and Dietetic, 11*(6), 511–7.

Introduction

It is estimated that 70% of the television advertisements marketed towards children are for food, while only 20% of the television advertisements marketed towards adults focus on food. Of the 70% of the ads for children, 98% focus on the marketing of foods high in salt, sugar, and fat. In an effort to understand the relationship between television advertisements and children's food choices, Hitchings and Moynihan (1998) interviewed 44 children between the ages of 9 and 11. The sample included 21 boys and 23 girls from a variety of socioeconomic classes and both private and state schools in Britain. The researchers collected information from the children's 3-day food diaries and child and parental interviews. Spearman's rank-order correlation coefficient, a nonparametric

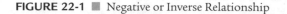

FIGURE 22-1 ■ Negative or Inverse Relationship

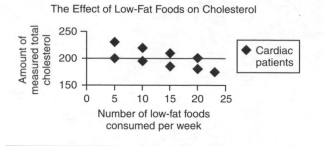

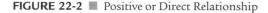

FIGURE 22-2 ■ Positive or Direct Relationship

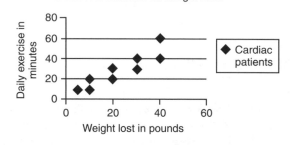

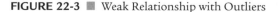

FIGURE 22-3 ■ Weak Relationship with Outliers

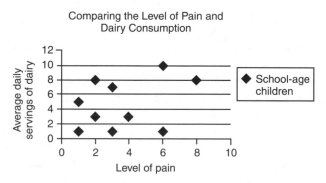

statistical analysis technique, was used to determine the relationship between the number of food advertisements remembered and the number of foods eaten. Results indicated that television advertisements are related to children's food choices.

Relevant Study Results

In Figure 1, Hitchings and Moynihan (1998) present the relationship between the number of food advertisements remembered and the number of foods eaten by 44 children. Children most frequently remembered foods from breakfast cereals; confectionery items including sweets, chocolate bars, chocolate biscuits, gum, and iced lollies; and soft drinks consisting of carbonated beverages, squashes, and fruit juices. Since these are foods common in Britain, think of biscuits as similar to cookies, iced lollies as comparable to popsicles, squashes as fruit drinks, and twiglets as a baked crispy snack similar to pretzels. Researchers found the strongest relationship between soft drinks ($r = 0.68$) and crisps (chips) and savory snacks, which included crisps, corn snacks, twiglets, nuts, popcorn, and savory biscuits ($r = 0.61$).

FIGURE 1 ■ Scatterplot illustrating the relationship between the number of food television advertisements which were remembered and the number of these foods which are subsequently eaten, for 44 children aged 10 years. (Hitchings, E., & Moynihan, P. J. (1998). The relationship between television food advertisements recalled and actual foods consumed by children. *Journal of Human Nutrition and Dietetics, 11*(6), p. 515.)

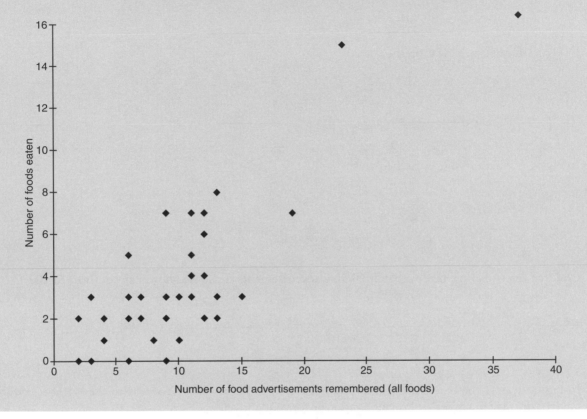

■ STUDY QUESTIONS

1. What type of relationship does Figure 22-1 illustrate? Provide a rationale for your answer.

2. By looking at the scatterplot shown in Figure 22-1, can you tell if the relationship is strong, moderate, or weak? Provide a rationale for your answer.

3. What is the strength of the relationship presented in Figure 22-3? Does this scatterplot have outliers? Provide a rationale for your answer.

4. In Figure 1, what variable is on the *x*-axis?

5. In Figure 1, what variable is on the *y*-axis?

6. Children remembering approximately 20 food advertisements consumed how many of those foods?

7. In Figure 1, does the Number of foods eaten positively or negatively correlate with the Number of food advertisements remembered? Provide a rationale for your answer.

8. Researchers found the strongest relationship between soft drinks and crisps. What was that relationship?

9. What information does Figure 1 of the study provide you about the influence of television food advertisements?

10. Should the results of this study be generalized to other countries? Provide a rationale for your answer.

◼ ANSWERS TO STUDY QUESTIONS

1. Figure 22-1 shows an inverse or negative relationship between the number of low-fat foods consumed per week and the amount of measured total cholesterol. The plotted points move from the left upper corner to the right lower corner, indicating a negative relationship.

2. Yes, by looking at a scatterplot you can tell whether the relationship is strong, moderate, or weak based on the closeness of the plotted points and if the points form a straight line. Thus, Figure 22-1 demonstrates a strong relationship based on the closeness of the points and the fairly straight line formed by the points that extends from the left upper corner of the graph to the right lower corner. The scatterplot shows the subjects' scores for the *x*-axis and *y*-axis and demonstrates the strong negative relationship between the number of low-fat foods consumed per week and the amount of measured total cholesterol.

3. Figure 22-3 illustrates a very weak relationship since the plotted points are spread out and do not form any type of straight line. Thus there is a very weak or really no relationship between level of pain and average daily servings of dairy. One would expect that these two variables are not related. The scatterplot also has two outliers with values very different from the other values.

4. In Figure 1, Number of food advertisements remembered (all foods) is placed on the *x* or the horizontal axis

5. In Figure 1, Number of foods eaten is placed on the *y* or vertical axis.

6. In Figure 1, children remembering approximately 20 foods consumed approximately 7 of those remembered.

7. The number of foods eaten positively correlates with the number of food advertisements remembered. Thus, the plotted points extend from the left lower corner to the right upper corner. Figure 1 shows the greater the number of food advertisements remembered, the greater the number of those foods that are eaten. Thus, the two variables vary together in the same direction, which indicates a positive or direct relationship.

8. The correlation between soft drinks and crisps was $r = 0.68$, which is included in the Relevant Study Results from the research article.

9. The relationship shown in Figure 1 indicates that television food advertisements do influence children's food choices. According to the study findings, children request food based on their remembrance of specific food advertisements on television. The children remembered the foods that are high in sugar, fats, and salt, which lack quality nutrition and could lead to weight gain.

10. Answers may vary. Although this study has identified a relationship between television viewing and foods eaten, the results of this study should not be generalized to other countries. For example, marketing strategies and target markets may differ in the United States, and this study specifically focused only on children aged 9–11 and foods high in salt, sugar, and fat. This study also has a small sample size of 44 subjects, which decreases the ability to generalize the study results. However, this study could be replicated to possibly establish similar trends in the United States and other countries for future generalization to other populations. Future studies should address children of all ages, the timing of the advertisement, and all types of food advertised, both healthy and unhealthy. However, many television advertisements focus more on sweets, chips, and high-calorie drinks than healthy food.

■ EXERCISE 22   Questions to be Graded

1. Why might a researcher choose to include a scatterplot in the publication of a study?

2. What type of relationship does Figure 22-2 illustrate? Provide a rationale for your answer.

3. Examine Figure 1 from the Hitchings and Moynihan (1998) study. Which category has a stronger relationship: the Less than 10 food advertisements remembered and the Number of foods eaten, or the More than 10 food advertisements remembered and the Number of foods eaten? Provide a rationale for your answer.

4. In Figure 1, children who remembered approximately 25 food advertisements consumed what number of foods?

5. Describe the pattern of plotted points in Figure 1 between Number of food advertisements remembered and Number of foods eaten. Include the direction and approximate strength of the relationship shown in the figure in your description.

6. What is an outlier? What are the ways in which an outlier might occur in a study?

7. Does Figure 1 from the Hitchings and Moynihan (1998) study have any outliers? Provide a rationale for your answer.

8. Researchers stated that 96% of food requests from the children were granted by their parents. How does this contribute to the hypothesis of the number of food advertisements remembered influencing the number of foods eaten? Provide a rationale for your answer.

9. According to the authors, studies conducted in the United States indicated a relationship between television and obesity. If television advertisements are related to children's food choices, what changes can the media make to promote a healthy diet in children? Provide a rationale for your answer.

10. Examine the scatterplots from this exercise, and then provide your own example of both negative and positive relationships in scatterplots.

PEARSON'S PRODUCT-MOMENT CORRELATION COEFFICIENT

STATISTICAL TECHNIQUE IN REVIEW

Many studies are conducted to identify relationships between or among variables. The correlational coefficient is the mathematical expression of the relationship studied. Three common analysis techniques are used to examine relationships: Spearman Rank-Order Correlation or *rho*, Kendall's Tau or *tau*, and the Pearson's Product-Moment Correlation Coefficient or *r*. Spearman and Kendall's Tau are used to examine relationships with ordinal level data. **Pearson's Correlation Coefficient** is the most common correlational analysis technique used to examine the relationship between two variables measured at the interval or ratio level.

Relationships are discussed in terms of direction and strength. The direction of the relationship is expressed as either positive or negative. A **positive or direct relationship** exists when one variable increases as does the other variable increases, or when one variable decreases as the other decreases. Conversely, a **negative or inverse relationship** exists when one variable increases and the other variable decreases. The strength of a relationship is described as weak, moderate, or strong. Pearson's *r* is never greater than -1.00 or $+1.00$, so an *r* value of -1.00 or $+1.00$ indicates the strongest possible relationship, either negative or positive, respectively. An *r* value of 0.00 indicates no relationship. To describe a relationship, the labels **weak ($r < 0.3$)**, **moderate ($r = 0.3$ to 0.5)**, and **strong ($r > 0.5$)** are used in conjunction with both positive and negative values of *r*. Thus, the strength of the negative relationships would be weak with $r < -0.3$, moderate with $r = -0.3$ to -0.5, and strong with $r > -0.5$ (Burns & Grove, 2007).

RESEARCH ARTICLE

Source: Keays, S. L., Bullock-Saxton, J. E., Newcombe, P., & Keays, A. C. (2003). The relationship between knee strength and functional stability before and after anterior cruciate ligament reconstruction. *Journal of Orthopedic Research, 21*(2), 231–7.

Introduction

Keays et al. (2003) conducted a correlational study to determine "the relationship between muscle strength and functional stability in 31 patients pre- and postoperatively, following a unilateral anterior cruciate ligament rupture" (Keays et al., 2003, p. 231). The results of the study showed a significant positive correlation between quadriceps strength indices and functional stability, both before and after surgery. No significant relationship was demonstrated between hamstring strength indices 60°/s and functional stability, as presented in Table 5.

Relevant Study Results

"Patients with an unstable knee as a result of an anterior cruciate ligament (ACL) rupture rely heavily on muscle function around the joint to maintain dynamic stability during functional activity. It is uncertain which muscles play the decisive role in functional stability or exactly which aspect of muscle function is most critical" (Keays et al., 2003, p. 231). "The aim of this study was to assess the relationship between muscle strength and functional stability of 31 patients pre- and postoperatively, following unilateral ACL ligament rupture" (Keays et al., 2003, p. 231). "To assess the relationship between maximum isokinetic strength and functional performance Pearson's correlations (r) were computed. . . . Due to the number of correlations computed, and therefore the increased likelihood that chance results may be evident, a more conservative significance level of $\alpha = 0.01$ was adopted to control for increased Type 1 error" (see Table 5; Keays et al., 2003, pp. 232–3).

TABLE 5 ■ Pearson's Product-Moment Correlation between Strength Indices and Function after Surgery					
	n	Quadriceps Strength Index 60°/s	Hamstring Strength Index 60°/s	Quadriceps Strength Index 120°/s	Hamstring Strength Index 20°/s
Hop index	31	$r = 0.655**$	$r = 0.247$	$r = 0.744**$	$r = 0.431*$
Sig. (two tailed)		$p = 0.000$	$p = 0.080$	$p = 0.000$	$p = 0.016$
Triple hop index	31	$r = 0.619**$	$r = 0.342$	$r = 0.742**$	$r = 0.420*$
Sig. (two tailed)		$p = 0.000$	$p = 0.060$	$p = 0.000$	$p = 0.019$
Shuttle run test	31	$r = -0.498**$	$r = -0.149$	$r = -0.457**$	$r = -0.178$
Sig. (two tailed)		$p = 0.004$	$p = 0.424$	$p = 0.010$	$p = 0.338$
Side step test	31	$r = -0.528**$	$r = -0.124$	$r = -0.519**$	$r = 0.238*$
Sig. (two tailed)		$p = 0.002$	$p = 0.506$	$p = 0.003$	$p = 0.198$
Carioca test	31	$r = -0.474*$	$r = -0.047$	$r = -0.510**$	$r = 0.267$
Sig. (two tailed)		$p = 0.000$	$p = 0.802$	$p = 0.003$	$p = 0.146$

*Correlation is significant at the 0.05 level (two tailed).
**Correlation is significant at the 0.01 level (two tailed).
Keays, S. L., Bullock-Saxton, J. E., Newcombe, P., & Keays, A. C. (2003). The relationship between knee strength and functional stability before and after anterior cruciate ligament reconstruction. *Journal of Orthopaedic Research, 21*(2), 235. Copyright © 2003, with permission from The Orthopaedic Research Society.

■ STUDY QUESTIONS

1. What is the value of the Pearson *r* for the relationship between the Hamstring strength index 120°/s and the Triple hop index?

2. What is the value of the Pearson *r* for the relationship between the Quadriceps strength index 120°/s and the Side step test? Is this *r* value significant?

3. The closer the value of r to 0.00 the stronger the relationship in a study. Is this statement true or false? Provide a rationale for your answer.

4. What values for r indicate the strongest possible relationships? What do those values also indicate?

5. Without using numbers, describe the relationship between the Quadriceps strength index 60°/s and the Hop index.

6. Describe the direction and strength of the relationship between the Quadriceps strength index 60°/s and the Triple hop index.

7. Which variable has the strongest relationship with the Hamstring strength index 60°/s? Explain the basis for your answer. Is this r value significant?

8. Which of the following sets of variables has the weakest relationship?
   a. Quadriceps strength index 60°/s and the Triple hop index
   b. Hamstring strength index 60°/s and the Carioca test
   c. Hamstring strength index 120°/s and the Side step test
   d. Quadriceps strength index 120°/s and the Shuttle run test

9. Can the Pearson r prove causality between variables? Provide a rationale for your answer.

10. Consider $r = -0.72$ and $r = -.72$. Describe any differences or similarities between these r values.

ANSWERS TO STUDY QUESTIONS

1. $r = 0.420$. The r value is listed in Table 5 for the relationship between the Hamstring strength index 120°/s and the Triple hop index.

2. $r = -0.519^{**}$. The r value is listed in Table 5 for the relationship between the Quadriceps strength index 120°/s and the Side step test. The ** indicate that the r value is statistically significant since its probability or $p = 0.003$, which is smaller than the significance level set at 0.01. The ** indicate the level of significance that is identified in the key below Table 5.

3. False. An r value of 0.00 indicates no relationship exists, so the closer the r value is to zero, the smaller the relationship.

4. The r values of +1.00 and –1.00 both indicate the strongest possible relationships among variables. Positive (+) 1.00 is the strongest or perfect positive relationship and indicates that variables change together, either increasing or decreasing simultaneously. Negative (–) 1.00 is the strongest or perfect negative relationship and indicates that variables change in opposite directions: as one variable increases another variable decreases. These extreme values are not found in studies since no variables have perfect positive or negative relationships.

5. $r = 0.655^{**}$. The r value listed for the Quadriceps strength index 60°/s and the Hop index indicates a strong, positive relationship, where the Quadriceps strength index 60°/s increases as the Hop index increases. Also, the relationship is significant at $p < 0.000$, and this p value is less than $\alpha = 0.01$, so the r value is statistically significant.

6. The relationship between the Quadriceps strength index 60°/s and the Triple hop index is $r = 0.619^{**}$. A positive or direct relationship exists between these two variables, indicating that the Quadriceps strength and Triple hop indices either increase or decrease together. This is a strong relationship since the $r > 0.5$. The r value is also statistically significant since $p = 0.000$ and this p value is less than $\alpha = 0.01$.

7. The Triple hop index has the strongest relationship with the Hamstring strength index 60°/s with an $r = 0.342$. Recall that the closer the value of r to 1.00 or –1.00, the stronger the relationship being described. This relationship is not significant since it has probability or $p = 0.060$ and this value is greater than $\alpha = 0.01$.

8. b. Hamstring strength index 60°/s and the Carioca test. The weakest relationship is between the Hamstring strength index of 60°/s and the Carioca test with an $r = -0.047$. The Answers a, c, and d had r values of 0.619, 0.238, and –0.457, respectively. Answer b is correct as its r value is the closest to 0.00.

9. The Pearson r does not prove causality between variables; it merely explains the strength and direction of the relationship between two variables. Relationships indicate that two variables are linked to each other but not that one variable brings about or causes the other. Causality indicates a strong relationship between two variables, but one of the variables must always precede the other in time and be present when the effect occurs. With causality, you manipulate the independent variable to create an effect on the dependent variable.

10. Both r values ($r = -0.72$ and $r = -.72$) have the same mathematical meaning, signifying a strong, negative relationship between two variables. Researchers are trending toward dropping the leading zeros before decimal points. Clinically, it has become important to use a leading zero prior to decimal points. In fact, the Joint Commission on Healthcare Organizations has mandated that the leading zero be present before decimals to alert the health care professional that the number is a decimal. Following this in clinical practice decreases the number of medication errors made.

Name: _____ Class: _____

Date: _____

■ EXERCISE 23 Questions to be Graded

1. What is the *r* value for the relationship between Hamstring strength index 60°/s and the Shuttle run test? Is this *r* value significant? Provide a rationale for your answer.

2. Consider *r* = 1.00 and *r* = –1.00. Which *r* value is stronger? Provide a rationale for your answer.

3. Describe the direction of the relationship between the Hamstring strength index 60°/s and the Shuttle run test.

4. Without using numbers, describe the relationship between the Hamstring strength index 120°/s and the Triple hop index.

5. Which variable has the weakest relationship with the Quadriceps strength index 120°/s? Provide a rationale for your answer.

6. Which of the following sets of variables has the strongest relationship?
   a. Hamstring strength index 120°/s and the Hop index
   b. Quadriceps strength index 60°/s and the Carioca test
   c. Quadriceps strength index 120°/s and the Side step test
   d. Quadriceps strength index 60°/s and the Triple hop index

7. In Table 5, two r values are reported as $r = -0.498$ and $r = -0.528$. Describe each r value in words, indicating which would be more statistically significant, and provide a rationale for your answer.

8. The researchers stated that the study showed a positive, significant correlation between Quadriceps strength indices and pre- and postoperative functional stability. Considering the data presented in the Table 5, do you agree with their statement? Provide a rationale for your answer.

9. The researchers stated that no significant relationship could be described between Hamstring strength indices 60°/s and functional stability. Given the data in Table 5, explain why not.

10. Consider the relationship reported for the Quadriceps strength index 120°/s and the Hop index ($r = 0.744^{**}$, $p = 0.000$). What do these r and p values indicate related to statistical significance and clinical importance?

24

UNDERSTANDING PEARSON'S r, EFFECT SIZE, AND PERCENTAGE OF VARIANCE EXPLAINED

STATISTICAL TECHNIQUE IN REVIEW

Review the statistical information regarding Pearson's Product-Moment Correlation Coefficient presented in Exercise 23. In this exercise, you will need to apply that information to gain an understanding of interpreting Pearson r results presented in a mirror-image table. A mirror-image table, as the name implies, has the same labels in the same order for both the x- and y-axes. Frequently, letters or numbers are assigned to each label, and only the letter or number designator is used to label one of the axes. To find the r value for a pair of variables, look both along the labeled or y-axis in the table below and then along the x-axis, using the letter designator assigned to the variable you want to know the relationship for, and find the cell in the table with the r value. Below is an example of a mirror-image table that compares hours of class attended, hours studying, and final grade as a percentage. The results in the table are intended as an example of a mirror-image table and are not based on research. If you were asked to identify the r value for the relationship between hours of class attended and the final grade as a percentage, the answer would be $r = 0.72$, and between hours studying and final grade as a percentage, the answer would be $r = 0.78$. The dash (–) marks located on the diagonal line of the table represent the variable's correlation with itself, which is always a perfect positive correlation or $r = +1.00$.

VARIABLES	A	B	C
A. Hours of class attended	–	0.44	0.72
B. Hours studying	0.44	–	0.78
C. Final grade as a percentage	0.72	0.78	–

Effect Size of an r Value

In determining the strength of a relationship, remember that a weak relationship is $r < 0.3$ or $r < -0.3$, a moderate relationship is $r = 0.3$ to 0.5 or -0.3 to -0.5, and a strong relationship is $r > 0.5$ or > -0.5. The r value is equal to the effect size or the strength of a relationship. In the table above, the relationship between hours of class attended and hours of studying is $r = 0.44$ and the effect size $= 0.44$. The effect size is used in power analysis to determine sample size for future studies. The strength of the effect size is the same as that for the r values, with a **weak effect size < 0.3 or < −0.3, a moderate effect size 0.3 to 0.5 or −0.3 to −0.5, and a strong effect size > 0.5 or > −0.5**. The smaller the effect size, the greater the sample size needed to detect significant relationships in future studies. Thus the larger the effect size, the smaller the sample size that is needed to determine significant relationships. The determination of study sample sizes with power analysis is presented in Exercise 12.

Percentage of Variance Explained in a Relationship

Percentage of variance explained is a calculation based on a Pearson's *r* value. The purpose for calculating the percentage of variance explained is to understand further the relationship or correlation between two variables in terms of clinical importance. To calculate the percentage of variance explained, square the *r* value then multiply by 100 to determine a percentage.

Formula: $r^2 \times 100$ = % variance explained
Example: $r = 0.78$ (correlation between hours studying and final grade as a percentage)
            $(0.78)^2 \times 100 = 0.6084 \times 100 = 60.84\%$ variance explained

The example above indicates that the hours studying can be used to predict 60.84% of the variance in the final course grade. Calculating the percentage of variance explained helps the researchers and consumers of research better understand the practical implications of reported results. The stronger the *r* value, the greater the percentage of variance explained. For example if $r = 0.5$, then 25% of the variance in one variable is explained by an another variable and if $r = 0.6$, then 36% of the variance is explained. Any Pearson's $r \geq 0.3$, which yields a 9% variance explained, is considered clinically important. Keep in mind that a result may be statistically significant ($p < 0.05$), but it may not represent a clinically important finding (Burns & Grove, 2005).

RESEARCH ARTICLE

Source: Hatchett, G. T., & Park, H. L. (2004). Relationships among optimism, coping styles, psychopathology, and counseling outcome. *Personality and Individual Differences, 36*(8), 1755–69.

Introduction

Hatchett and Park (2004) conducted a study consisting of 96 college students to determine the relationships between optimism, coping styles, psychopathology, and counseling outcomes. Each participant filled out three questionnaires before beginning counseling: the Outcome Questionnnaire-45 (OQ-45) (measures psychopathology), the Life Orientation Test-Revised (LOT-R) (measures optimism and pessimism), and the Coping Inventory for Stressful Situations (CISS) (measures coping styles). At the termination of treatment, the OQ-45 was re-administered. The researchers reported that optimism "was negatively correlated with psychopathology, emotion-oriented coping, and the avoidance-distraction subscale from the CISS" (Hatchett & Park, 2004, p. 1762). Conversely, they report optimism to be positively correlated with task-oriented coping and the avoidance–social diversion subscales. Pessimism reportedly had the opposite or negative relationships with these same variables. The researchers reported no statistically significant correlation between optimism and counseling outcomes. "Future research might be directed at determining whether the early assessment and subsequent remediation of pessimistic thoughts leads to better outcomes. Furthermore research might ascertain whether optimists and pessimists respond differently to certain types of clinical interventions. [One] might advocate matching clinical interventions to clients' unique personality characteristics. For example, optimists, who rely more on problem-focused coping strategies, might respond better to more active intervention strategies (e.g., problem-solving skills). On the other hand, pessimists, who report greater use of emotion-oriented coping, might respond better to more expressive and supportive therapeutic techniques" (Hatchett & Park, 2004, pp. 1766–7).

Relevant Study Results

In Table 2 in p. 175, Hatchett and Park (2004) presented the correlations among optimism (LOT-R Total and Positive Items); pessimism (Negative Items); psychopathology (OQ-45); and coping styles (Task, Emotion, Avoidance, Avoidance–Distraction, and Avoidance–Social Diversion). Table 2 is a mirror-image table with the variables numbered and labeled on the *y*-axis and the numbers of the variables on the *x*-axis. The blank spaces in the table are where the variable is correlated with itself and would be a +1.00 correlation.

TABLE 2 ■ Intercorrelations among Optimism, Psychopathology, and Coping Styles									
Variable	1	2	3	4	5	6	7	8	9
1. OQ-45 (psychopathology)	–	–0.72**	–0.59**	0.74**	–0.43**	0.76**	–0.22*	0.09	–0.45**
2. LOT-R Total (optimism)		–	0.92**	–0.94**	0.54**	–0.58**	0.11	–0.20*	0.38**
3. Positive Items (from LOT-R)			–	–0.72**	0.53**	–0.48**	0.15	–0.16	0.38**
4. Negative Items (from LOT-R)				–	–0.47**	0.58**	–0.06	0.21*	–0.32**
5. Task (coping style)					–	–0.42**	0.08	–0.09	0.22*
6. Emotion (coping style)						–	–0.02	0.21*	–0.24*
7. Avoidance (coping style)							–	0.83**	0.78**
8. Avoidance-Distraction (coping style)								–	0.36**
9. Avoidance-Social Diversion (coping style)									–

*$p < 0.05$.
**$p < 0.01$.
Hatchett, G. T., & Park, H. L. (2003). Relationships among optimism, coping styles, psychopathology, and counseling outcome. *Personality and Individual Differences, 36*(8), p. 1762. Copyright © 2003, with permission from Elsevier.

■ STUDY QUESTIONS

1. In Table 2, what is the numeric value given for the correlation between LOT-R Total and Negative Items?

2. Describe the correlation in Question 1 using words. Is this relationship statistically significant? Provide a rationale for your answer.

3. Calculate the percentage of variance explained by the relationship of OQ-45 or psychopathology and Task coping style. Is this correlation clinically important? Is the correlation statistically significant? Provide a rationale for your answers.

4. Which two variables in Table 2 have the strongest correlation? Provide a rationale for your answer.

5. Is the correlation between Emotion coping style and OQ-45 or psychopathology scores statistically significant? Is it clinically important? Provide a rationale for your answers.

6. As a clinician, does knowledge of the correlation in Question 5 enhance your practice? Provide a rationale for your answer.

7. What is the effect size of the relationship between variables 3 and 8? Describe the strength of this effect size. What is the value of knowing the effect size? Discuss the percentage of variance explained by this relationship.

8. Consider two values, $r = -0.24$ and $r = 0.78$. How would you describe them in relationship to each other?

9. Compare the percentages of variance explained for the *r* values in Question 8.

10. What *r* value would you expect to have been recorded in place of each dash (–) had the researchers chosen to record a number? Provide a rationale for your answer.

ANSWERS TO STUDY QUESTIONS

1. $r = -0.94^{**}$, $p < 0.01$ is the correlation between LOT-R Total and Negative Items.

2. $r = -0.94^{**}$ represents a strong, negative relationship between LOT-R (optimism) and Negative Items; therefore, as LOT-R values or optimism increase, the values of the Negative Items decrease. This *r* value has ** next to it, so it is statistically significant at $p < 0.01$, as indicated by the key below the table.

3. The correlation between OQ-45 or psychopathology and Task coping style is $r = -0.43^{**}$.

    Percentage of variance = $r^2 \times 100$ Percentage of variance = $(-0.43)^2 \times 100 = 18.49\%$

    The relationship represented by $r = -0.43$ is clinically important. Scores on the OQ-45 questionnaire measuring psychopathology can be used to explain 18.49% of the variance in the Task coping style scores. The $r = -0.43^{**}$ is also statistically significant at $p < 0.01$ (see the key at the bottom of Table 2).

4. LOT-R Total (optimism) and Negative Items have the strongest relationship with $r = -0.94^{**}$. This *r* value is the closest to -1 and the farthest value from 0.00, which indicates it is the strongest relationship in the table. The relationship is significant at $p < 0.01$ as indicated by **.

5. $r = 0.76^{**}$ indicates the *r* value is statistically significant at $p < 0.01$ as indicated by the key below Table 2. Percentage of variance = $r^2 \times 100 = (0.76)^2 \times 100 = 57.76\%$. This correlation is clinically important with a percentage of variance greater than 9% and is actually 57.76%, indicating that the OQ-45 scores can be used to predict 57.76% of the variance in the Emotion coping style scores.

6. Knowing that scores on the psychopathology scale, OQ-45, allows the prediction of 57.76% of the variance in the emotion-based coping style scores. Thus, knowing the scores on one scale can allow prediction of scores on another scale, and that would be helpful to practicing professionals who might have time to administer one scale but not both. So the scores on the psychopathology scale provide understanding and prediction of the scores on the emotion-based coping style scale.

7. $r = -0.16$ is also the effect size. The effect size is negative and small for the relationship between positive items and avoidance-distraction coping style. The effect size is used in the calculation of a power analysis to determine sample size for future studies. Percentage of variance = $(-0.16)^2 \times 100 = 2.56\%$. The positive items scores can only predict 2.56% of the variance in avoidance-distraction coping style scores, so this is clinically not a very important relationship due to its weak effect size and small percentage of variance explained.

8. $r = 0.78$ is a strong positive relationship and is the stronger relationship of the two, as $r = -0.24$ indicates a weak negative relationship. The *r* value closest to 0.00 is considered the weakest relationship. Also, $r = 0.78^{**}$ is more significant at $p < 0.01$, where $r = -0.24^*$ is significant at $p < 0.05$. The smaller the *p* value, the more significant the result.

9. The percentage of variance explained for $r = 0.78$ is $(0.78)^2 \times 100 = 60.84\%$. The percentage of variance explained for $r = -0.24$ is $(-0.24)^2 \times 100 = 5.76\%$. Thus, the first relationship is much more useful in clinical practice in understanding the relationship between two variables, since 60.84% of the variance is explained with this relationship versus 5.76% by the second relationship. Recall that percentage of variance >9% indicates clinical importance.

10. $r = 1.00$. The dash recorded on each line forms a diagonal line across Table 2 where each item would be correlated with itself [e.g., 2. LOT-R Total with 2.(LOT-R Total)]. The relationship of an item with itself is always a perfect positive correlation, or $r = +1.00$.

■ EXERCISE 24   Questions to Be Graded

1. What is the *r* value listed for the relationship between variables 4 and 9?

2. Describe the correlation $r = -0.32^{**}$ using words. Is this a statistically significant correlation? Provide a rationale for your answer.

3. Calculate the percentage of variance explained for $r = 0.53$. Is this correlation clinically important? Provide a rationale for your answer.

4. According to Table 2, $r = 0.15$ is listed as the correlation between which two items? Describe this relationship. What is the effect size for this relationship, and what size sample would be needed to detect this relationship in future studies?

5. Calculate the percentage of variance explained for $r = 0.15$. Describe the clinical importance of this relationship.

6. Which two variables in Table 2, have the weakest correlation, or *r* value? Which relationship is the closest to this *r* value? Provide a rationale for your answer.

7. Is the correlation between LOT-R Total scores and Avoidance-Distraction coping style statistically significant? Is this relationship relevant to practice? Provide rationales for your answers.

8. Is the correlation between variables 9 and 4 significant? Is this correlation relevant to practice? Provide a rationale for your answer.

9. Consider two values, $r = 0.08$ and $r = -0.58$. Describe them in relationship to each other. Describe the clinical importance of both *r* values.

10. Examine the Pearson *r* values for LOT-R Total, which measured Optimism with the Task and Emotion Coping Styles. What do these results indicate? How might you use this information in your practice?

■ BONUS QUESTION

One of the study goals was to examine the relationship between optimism and psychopathology. Using the data in Table 2, formulate an opinion regarding the overall correlation between optimism and psychopathology. Provide a rationale for your answer.

MULTIPLE CORRELATIONS I

STATISTICAL TECHNIQUE IN REVIEW

There are times when more than one variable is used to predict the outcome of another variable. This is referred to as multiple correlations. A series of Pearson r values are calculated to determine the relationship among those variables. The results of the Pearson r values are then inserted into another formula, which produces the multiple correlation coefficient or R. The R represents the extent to which the independent variables predict the outcome of the dependant or outcome variable. Another term for the outcome variable is the *criterion variable*. An example used to explain multiple correlations is the use of high school grade point average (GPA) and SAT scores to predict college GPA. The number that is represented by the r value tells us the strength of the relationship between the variables. For example, r values of < 0.3 or < -0.3 represent weak linear relationships, r values of 0.3 to 0.5 or -0.3 to -0.5 are moderate linear relationships, and r values > 0.5 or >-0.5 represent strong linear relationships (Burns & Grove, 2005). Review Exercises 23 and 24 if you have questions about correlations.

RESEARCH ARTICLE

Source: Abbasi, R., Brown, B. W., Lamendola, C., McLaughlin, T., & Reaven, G. M. (2002). Relationship between obesity, insulin resistance, and coronary heart disease risk. *Journal of the American College of Cardiology, 40*(5), 937–43.

Introduction

A study was conducted by Abbasi et al. (2002) to examine the relationship between body mass index (BMI) and insulin resistance, and to determine the relationship between these two variables and coronary heart disease (CHD) risk factors. The study sample consisted of 314 volunteers who were nondiabetic, normotensive, and healthy. The participants were 77% Caucasian, 12% Asian, 10% Hispanic, and 1% African American. The researchers found that BMI and steady-state plasma glucose (SSPG), which is a measure of insulin resistance, were significantly related to the risk factors of CHD. Thus, the researchers concluded that "obesity and insulin resistance are both powerful predictors of CHD risk, and insulin resistance at any given degree of obesity accentuates the risk of CHD and type 2 diabetes" (Abbasi et al., 2002, p. 937).

Relevant Study Results

The subjects' BMI was calculated, and fasting plasma glucose and insulin concentration were measured before, during, and after the ingestion of 75g of oral glucose. Insulin-mediated glucose disposal was also estimated by an insulin suppression test.

The sample was divided into three categories according to BMI, with each group having similar age and gender distributions. When comparing BMI and SSPG, the researchers found that the greater the SSPG concentration, the higher the BMI category. The SSPG values varied within the BMI range and 25% of the insulin-resistant individuals were in the normal weight category.

Simple and partial correlation coefficients between each of the CHD risk factors and BMI, and the CHD risk factors and SSPG are presented in Table 2. The partial correlation coefficients represent the results when adjusted for gender. Multiple regression analysis of the relationship between the CHD risk factors with BMI and SSPG jointly, with and without an interaction term, are represented in Table 3. Standardized regression coefficients are also recorded in Table 2 and are represented by β (Abbasi et al., 2002).

TABLE 2 ■ Simple and Partial Correlation Coefficients (*r*) between Coronary Heart Disease Risk Factors, BMI, and SSPG

Risk Factors	BMI		SSPG	
	Simple	Partial	Simple	Partial
Age	0.189*	0.180*	0.106†	0.113*
SBP	0.286	0.278	0.160*	0.168*
DBP	0.139*	0.125*	0.202	0.216
Total cholesterol	0.348	0.349	0.242	0.243
TG	0.444	0.437	0.507	0.520
HDL cholesterol	−0.385	−0.382	−0.410	−0.461
LDL cholesterol	0.361	0.355	0.223	0.229
Glucose response	0.306	0.303	0.573	0.577
Insulin response	0.380	0.379	0.630	0.631

Partial correlation coefficients were calculated after adjusting for differences in gender; all *p* values are < 0.001 except for *p < 0.05 and †*p* = 0.16. BMI = body mass index; DBP = diastolic blood pressure; HDL = high-density cholesterol; LDL = low-density cholesterol; SBP = systolic blood pressure; SSPG = steady-state plasma glucose; TG = triglycerides.

Abbasi, R., Brown, B. W., Lamendola, C., McLaughlin, T., & Reaven, G. M. (2002). Relationship between obesity, insulin resistance, and coronary heart disease risk. *Journal of the American College of Cardiology, 40*(5), p. 939. Copyright © 2002, with permission from The American College of Cardiology Foundation.

TABLE 3 ■ Multiple Regression Analysis of the Relationship between the CHD Risk Factors with BMI and SSPG Jointly, without an Interaction Term (Model A), and with the Interaction Term (Model B)

CHD Risk Factors	MODEL A		MODEL B		
	BMI	SSPG	BMI	SSPG	BMI × SSPG
Age	$R_A = 0.190$			$R_B = 0.190$	
B	0.178	0.023	0.183	0.043	−0.023
SE	0.215	0.012	0.428	0.076	0.003
P	0.005	0.711	0.145	0.915	0.961
SBP	$R_A = 0.288$			$R_B = 0.290$	
B	0.27	0.035	0.205	−0.207	0.280
SE	0.185	0.01	0.368	0.066	0.002
P	<0.001	0.573	0.094	0.601	0.537
DBP	$R_A = 0.208$			$R_B = 0.210$	
B	0.058	0.175	0.105	0.349	−0.202
SE	0.143	0.008	0.284	0.051	0.002
P	0.357	0.006	0.401	0.388	0.663
Total cholesterol	$R_A = 0.358$			$R_B = 0.359$	
B	0.301	0.098	0.244	−0.103	0.235
SE	0.561	0.032	1.115	0.198	0.007
P	<0.001	0.117	0.049	0.788	0.596
TG	$R_A = 0.556$			$R_B = 0.557$	
B	0.260	0.382	0.196	0.154	0.267
SE	0.860	0.049	1.709	0.302	0.011
P	<0.001	<0.001	0.077	0.655	0.501
HDL cholesterol	$R_A = -0.463$			$R_B = -0.477$	
B	−0.246	−0.293	−0.468	−1.08	0.922
SE	0.195	0.011	0.386	0.068	0.003
P	<0.001	<0.001	<0.001	0.003	0.029
LDL cholesterol	$R_A = 0.365$			$R_B = 0.366$	
B	0.330	0.065	0.347	0.128	−0.073
SE	0.505	0.029	1.009	0.179	0.007
P	<0.001	0.292	0.005	0.740	0.870
Glucose response	$R_A = 0.575$			$R_B = 0.584$	
B	0.051	0.549	−0.144	−0.171	0.836
SE	0.947	0.052	1.872	0.334	0.012
P	0.332	<0.001	0.165	0.609	0.030
Insulin response	$R_A = 0.638$			$R_B = 0.649$	
B	0.110	0.579	−0.123	−0.283	0.999
SE	1.628	0.090	3.203	0.571	0.021
P	0.026	<0.001	0.208	0.368	0.006

β = standardized regression coefficient; BMI = body mass index; CHD = coronary-heart disease; DBP = diastolic blood pressure; HDL = high-density cholesterol; LDL = low-density cholesterol; R_A = multiple correlation coefficients for model A; R_B = multiple correlation coefficients for model B; SBP = systolic blood pressure; SSPG = steady-state plasma glucose; TG = triglycerides.

Abbasi, R., Brown, B. W., Lamendola, C., McLaughlin, T., & Reaven, G. M. (2002). Relationship between obesity, insulin resistance, and coronary heart disease risk. *Journal of the American College of Cardiology, 40*(5), p. 940. Copyright © 2002, with permission from The American College of Cardiology Foundation.

■ STUDY QUESTIONS

1. Which correlation coefficient was higher for the risk factor of total cholesterol, BMI or SSPG? Provide a rationale for your answer.

2. Were the correlations higher for BMI or SSPG for the risk factor of age?

3. Examine all the relationships represented in Table 2 and identify the strongest correlation value. Explain why you think it is the strongest correlation between two variables.

4. Identify the type and strength of the relationship between HDL cholesterol and SSPG simple presented in Table 2.

5. In this study, which variable(s) is/are referred to as outcome or dependent variable(s)?

6. What are the results of the multiple regression analysis for age for Models A and B? What does this mean?

7. What are the results of the multiple regression analysis for glucose response for Models A and B?

8. What is the difference between Model A and Model B in Table 3? What does it mean?

9. Describe the statistical significance of the results presented in Table 2.

◼ ANSWERS TO STUDY QUESTIONS

1. Using Table 2, the BMI correlations were higher for total cholesterol with $r = 0.348$ for simple and $r = 0.349$ for partial correlation coefficients, versus 0.242 and 0.243 for SSPG.

2. Examining the results from Table 2, the correlations were higher for BMI. The simple correlation coefficient was $r = 0.189$ and the partial correlation coefficient was $r = 0.180$. For SSPG, the simple correlation was $r = 0.106$ and the partial correlation was $r = 0.113$.

3. Insulin response and SSPG partial correlation is the strongest relationship with $r = 0.631$. The correlation value closest to +1 or –1 represents the strongest relationship, since the closer the value is to +1 or –1 the stronger the correlation between two variables. A correlation value of $r = 1$ or $r = -1$ is a perfect relationship and $r = 0$ indicates no relationship between variables. A correlation value of $r = 0.631$ would be considered a strong relationship since it is >0.5.

4. The relationship between HDL cholesterol and SSPG Simple is $r = -0.410$. The type of relationship is negative, as HDL cholesterol increases SSPG decreases, and the strength of the relationship is moderate since the value is between –0.3 and –0.5.

5. The outcome or dependent variables for this study are coronary heart disease (CHD) risk factors (age, SBP, DBP, total cholesterol, TG, HDL cholesterol, LDL cholesterol, glucose response, and insulin response).

6. In Table 3, the multiple regression analysis Model A is $R_A = 0.190$, and for Model B the result is also $R_B = 0.190$. These values represent a weak relationship between age and BMI and age and SSPG. When looking at age compared with the other CHD risk factors, age is the number closest to 0 and is therefore the weakest relationship.

7. In Table 3, the multiple regression analysis result for glucose response using Model A is $R_A = 0.575$ and using Model B is $R_B = 0.584$.

8. Model A does not use the interaction term and Model B uses the interaction term. The interaction term represents the relationship between BMI and SSPG and takes into consideration that these two variables (BMI and SSPG) have an overlapping effect and are not completely independent of each other.

9. All the p values are <0.001, except for *$p < 0.05$ (age/BMI simple and partial, age/SSPG partial, SBP/SSPG simple and partial, and DBP/BMI simple and partial) and †$p = 0.16$ for age/SSPG simple; thus, the relationship $r = 0.106$† is the only nonsignificant correlation in Table 2.

Name: _____ Class: _____

Date: _____

■ EXERCISE 25 | Questions to be Graded

1. Which variable (BMI or SSPG) had a lower correlation with glucose response? Provide a rationale for your answer.

2. Which variable (BMI or SSPG) had higher correlations with systolic blood pressure? Provide a rationale for your answer.

3. Which result in Table 2 represents the weakest relationship? Provide a rationale for your answer.

4. What were the standardized regression coefficients for LDL cholesterol?

5. What were the standardized regression coefficients for insulin response?

6. The article states that the higher the BMI variable, the greater the SSPG. What does this tell you about the type of relationship between these two independent variables?

7. Were all of the insulin-resistant individuals obese?

8. The researchers used BMI as a measure of obesity. Name two other ways to measure body fat distributions.

9. A multiple correlation coefficient greater than 0.5 (>0.5) is a strong relationship between variables. In Table 3, identify the relationships that fall into the strong category and explain what these relationships might mean in clinical practice.

10. The majority of the participants in this study were Caucasian (77%). Does this change the way the information can be used in clinical practice? Can findings be generalized to populations of ethnically diverse patients? Provide a rationale for your answer.

26

MULTIPLE CORRELATIONS II

STATISTICAL TECHNIQUE IN REVIEW

In Exercise 25, we examined the multiple correlation coefficient (R). R is calculated when more than one variable is used to predict the outcome of another variable. When the multiple correlation coefficient (R) is squared, the result is referred to as the coefficient of determination or R^2. The coefficient of determination lets you know how much of the variance in the outcome or dependent variable is predicted by the independent or predictor variables. The coefficient of determination is usually written as a percentage. Thus an R^2 value of $0.45 \times 100\% = 45\%$, which means that 45% of the variation in the dependent variable is due to its dependence on the independent variables and can be predicted by the independent variables (Burns & Grove, 2005).

RESEARCH ARTICLE

Source: DeBourgh, G. A. (2003). Predictors of student satisfaction in distance-delivered graduate nursing courses: What matters most? *Journal of Professional Nursing, 19*(3), 149–63.

Introduction

DeBourgh (2003) investigated student satisfaction with a graduate level nursing course that was taught via interactive video teleconferencing (IVT) and the Internet. The 43 graduate students were enrolled in a nursing theory master's level course at a state university. All of the subjects were employed as nurses, with 56% of them working more than 39 hours each week. The results of the study were that the most important aspects of instruction in regard to student satisfaction were the quality and effectiveness of the instructor and the way that the instructor conveyed information.

Relevant Study Results

"The distance-education program that provided the research setting for this study used systems theory to show and operationalize the school's philosophy, mission, and conceptual model of nursing education and evaluation. . . . The predictor [or independent] variables of this study (learner attributes, technology, instructor/instruction, and course management) are placed in the transformation component of the system (i.e., the learning process) and the criterion [or dependent] variable (student satisfaction) is placed as the output of the system" (DeBourgh, 2003, p. 153). Using a correlational predictive design, the relationships between 5 learner attributes and the other 3 independent variables were examined. The 5 learner attributes were previous experience with courses taught via technology, self-rating of competence with technology, frequency of between-class usage of communications technology, age, and remote-site group size. Student satisfaction was measured via a 59-item Student Satisfaction Survey (SSS).

When calculating for simple correlation coefficients, the results directed the researchers to further calculate an intercorrelation matrix using the 17 survey questions within the facet of instructor/instruction in order to examine the relationship between those items and course satisfaction. When the Pearson's Product-Moment Correlations were computed with student satisfaction, only instructor/instruction was found to be statistically significant: $r = .46, p = .01$.

Stepwise regression was conducted in order to determine which of the 8 independent variables (5 learner attribute variables—previous technology courses, technology competence, between-class technology usage, age, and remote-site group size, and 3 instructional variables—instructor/instruction, technology, and course management) were the best predictors of student satisfaction. Instructor/instruction, which was the only independent variable to show statistical significance, was the first to be entered into the regression equation followed by the next two highest correlated independent variables, between class technology use and competence with technology. These results are represented in Table 3.

After constructing the intercorrelation matrix of the 17 satisfaction survey questions within the facet of instructor/instruction, it was found that "8 questions within this facet correlated strongly with the criterion [student satisfaction]: overall instructor rating ($r = .56, p = .01$); the promptness with which the instructor recognized and responded to students' questions ($r = .50, p = .01$); the instructor's professional behavior ($r = .39, p = .01$); the extent to which the instructor encouraged class participation ($r = .39, p = .05$); the clarity with which class assignments were communicated ($r = .56, p = .05$); the accessibility of the instructor outside of the class ($r = .36, p = .05$); instructional techniques that helped the understanding of course material ($r = .34, p = .05$); and the timeliness with which written work was graded and returned ($r = .33, p = .05$)" (DeBourgh, 2003. p. 156). Six of these 8 variables explained 38% of the total variance in student satisfaction. Stepwise multiple regression analysis of 6 of the survey questions is represented in Table 4.

TABLE 3 ■ Results of the Stepwise Multiple Regression Analysis Relating Student Satisfaction to Instructor/Instruction, Between-Class Use of Technology, and Competency with Technology for 43 Graduate Nurse Students

Step	Variable	R	R^2	R^2 Change	β	CUMULATIVE F	CUMULATIVE P
1	Instructor/instruction	.462	.213	.213	.952	11.12	.01*
2	Between-class technology use	.510	.261	.048	−.219	7.05	.12
3	Competence with technology	.512	.262	.001	.060	4.62	.78

*$P \leq .01$.
DeBourgh, G. A. (2003). Predictors of student satisfaction in distance-delivered graduate nursing courses: What matters most? *Journal of Professional Nursing, 19*(3), p. 156.

TABLE 4 ■ Results of the Stepwise Multiple Regression Analysis Relating Student Satisfaction to 6 Survey Questions within the Facet of Instructor/Instruction for 43 Graduate Nurse Students

Step	Variable	R	R^2	R^2 Change	β	CUMULATIVE F	CUMULATIVE P
1	Overall instructor rating	.557	.310	.310	.892	18.47	.01*
2	Instructor accessibility	.576	.332	.022	−.232	9.94	.26
3	Prompt response, question and answer	.599	.359	.027	.265	7.29	.20
4	Clarity of assignments	.607	.368	.009	.147	5.54	.46
5	Participation encouraged	.611	.373	.005	−.153	4.42	.58
6	Instructional techniques	.616	.380	.007	.160	3.67	.56

NOTE. Other survey questions did not enter the equation.
*$P \leq .01$.
DeBourgh, G. A. (2003). Predictors of student satisfaction in distance-delivered graduates nursing courses: What matters most? *Journal of Professional Nursing, 19*(3), p. 157.

"Potential limitations to the generalizability of the findings include the size and homogeneity of the study sample and the high quality of the technology used. The 43 subjects were highly experienced female nurses, employed full-time, self-motivated adults, in a self-selected intact group who were enrolled in a mandatory course that was available only via distance education. The study should be replicated using a larger sample and include undergraduate students to enhance generalizability" (DeBourgh, 2003, p. 158).

■ STUDY QUESTIONS

1. List the independent or predictor variables examined in the study.

2. Identify the dependent variable(s) in this study.

3. Which independent variable(s) showed a statistically significant relationship to student satisfaction? Provide a rationale for your answer.

4. What is the value of the multiple correlation coefficient (R) when instructor/instruction and between-class technology usage are added into the regression analysis?

5. What percent of the variance in student satisfaction is accounted for by instructor/instruction?

6. In Table 3, what is the difference in the predictive value of instructor/instruction only versus the 3 independent variables to predict student satisfaction? Examine the R and R^2 values as a basis for your response.

7. Based on the results presented in Table 3, what is the best predictor variable for student satisfaction? Provide a rationale for your response.

8. Competency with technology was not found to be a statistically significant predictor of student satisfaction. What are some possible reasons for this finding?

9. After initial review of the statistical results, the researchers conducted an additional analysis. What was this analysis, and why was it conducted?

■ ANSWERS TO STUDY QUESTIONS

1. The 8 independent or predictor variables consisted of 5 learner variables (previous experience with technology courses, technology competence, frequency of between-class usage of technology, age, and remote–site group size) and 3 instructional variables (instructor/instruction, technology, and course management).

2. The dependent variable in this study is student satisfaction. The overall student satisfaction was further broken down into overall satisfaction with the course and satisfaction with the course compared with conventional classroom courses.

3. Instructor/instruction was the only independent variable found to correlate significantly with the dependent variable student satisfaction, $r = .462$, $p = .01$.

4. The combination of instructor/instruction and between-class technology usage is $R = .510$. This value can be found in Table 3 and is the second step of the regression analysis. The multiple correlation value of $R = .510$ is the value of instructor/instruction and between-class technology usage to predict student satisfaction.

5. The answer is 21.3%. In Table 3 in the R^2 column, instructor/instruction has an $R^2 = .213$, which can be changed to a percent by the following computation: $0.213 \times 100\% = 21.3\%$

6. For the 3 independent variables in Table 3, the $R = .512$; and for instructor/instruction, $R = .462$, so there is a .05 difference between the two R values. In examining R^2, the difference between including instructor/instruction in the regression analysis is $R^2 = .213$ and including the 3 independent variables is $R^2 = .262$, or a difference of .049 or 4.9%. Thus, the results indicate that instructor/instruction provides the greatest prediction of student satisfaction, and the 3 independent variables only increase the predictive ability slightly (4.9%).

7. In this study, instructor/instruction is the best predictor of student satisfaction. Instructor/instruction has the only statistically significant correlation with student satisfaction, has the greatest $R = .462$, the largest $R^2 = .213$, and is significant with $F = 11.12$, $p = .01$.

8. The subjects chosen for this study were all masters' level registered nurses, who were working while attending school. Most clinical agencies require the use of computers by nurses, so they have basic computer skills. In addition, masters' students are self-motivated and goal-oriented and would ensure that they obtained the computer skills they needed to complete their graduate courses successfully.

9. The researchers found that the only independent variable significantly correlated with student satisfaction was instructor/instruction, so they conducted additional stepwise multiple regression analysis on the 6 survey questions for the facet of instructor/instruction to determine which of these were most predictive of student satisfaction. The results of this regression analysis are presented in Table 4.

■ EXERCISE 26   Questions to be Graded

1. For the facet of instructor/instruction, which response was found to be of statistical significance? Provide a rationale for your answer.

2. How much of the variance of student satisfaction within the facet of instructor/instruction is accounted for by the combination of overall instructor rating, instructor accessibility, and prompt response to questions and answers?

3. What is the multiple correlation coefficient (R) for overall instructor rating?

4. What is the multiple correlation coefficient (R) when the first 4 independent variables in Table 4 are included in the stepwise multiple regression analysis?

5. What percent of student satisfaction variance is explained by overall instructor rating?

6. What percent of student satisfaction variance can be accounted for when all 6 independent variables are included in the stepwise multiple regression analysis?

7. As you go down the *R* or multiple correlation column, the values increase. What does this mean?

8. Do these study results provide significant information about the use of distance technology for the delivery of courses to the general public?

9. This course was offered only through the Internet. How do you think this affected the study results? Did this strengthen the study?

10. In Table 3, one independent variable (instructor/instruction) was found to strongly predict the variance in student satisfaction. Was this result statistically significant? Was the result clinically significant? Provide rationales for your answers.

SIMPLE LINEAR REGRESSION

STATISTICAL TECHNIQUE IN REVIEW

Linear regression provides a means to estimate or predict the value of a dependent variable based on the value of one or more independent variables. The regression equation is a mathematical expression of a causal proposition emerging from a theoretical framework. The linkage between the theoretical statement and the equation is made prior to data collection and analysis. Linear regression is a statistical method of estimating the expected value of one variable, y, given the value of another variable, x. The term **simple linear regression** refers to the use of one independent variable, x, to predict one dependent variable, y.

The regression line is usually plotted on a graph, with the horizontal axis representing x (the independent or predictor variable) and the vertical axis representing the y (the dependent or predicted variable) (see Figure 27-1). The value represented by the letter a is referred to as the y intercept or the point where the regression line crosses or intercepts the y-axis. At this point on the regression line, $x = 0$. The value represented by the letter b is referred to as the slope, or the coefficient of x. The slope determines the direction and angle of the regression line within the graph. The slope expresses the extent to which y changes for every 1-unit change in x. The score on variable y (dependent variable) is predicted from the subject's known score on variable x (independent variable). The predicted score or estimate is referred to as $\hat{Y}$ (expressed as y-hat) (Burns & Grove, 2005).

FIGURE 27-1 ▨ Graph of a Simple Linear Regression Line

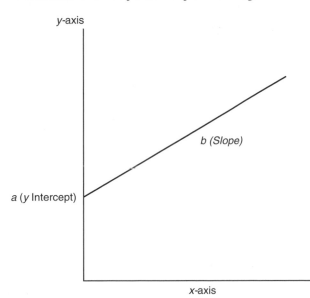

Simple linear regression is an effort to explain the dynamics within a scatter plot by drawing a straight line through the plotted scores. No single regression line can be used to predict with complete accuracy every y value from every x value. However, the purpose of the regression equation is to develop the line to allow the highest degree of prediction possible, the **line of best fit**. The procedure for developing the line of best fit is the **method of least squares**. If the data were perfectly correlated, all data points would fall along the straight line or line of best fit. However, not all data points fall on the line of best fit in studies, but the line of best fit provides the best equation for the values of y to be predicted by locating the intersection of points on the line for any given value of x.

The algebraic equation for the regression line of best fit is: $\hat{Y} = a + b$, where:
$\hat{Y}$ is the predicted value of y,
a is the y intercept and represents the value of y when $x = 0$ (see Figure 27-1),
a is also called the **regression constant**,
b is the slope of the line that is the amount of change in y for each one unit of change in x,
b is also called the **regression coefficient.**

In Figure 27-2, the x-axis represents Gestational Age and the y-axis represents Birth Weight. As gestational age increases from 20 weeks to 34 weeks, birth weight also increases. In other words, the slope of the line is positive. This line of best fit can be used to predict the birth weight (dependent variable) for an infant based on his or her gestational age in weeks (independent variable). Figure 27-2 is an example of a line of best fit and was not developed from research. In addition, the x-axis was started with 22 weeks rather than 0, which is the usual start in a regression figure. Using the formula $\hat{Y} = a + bx$, the birth weight of a baby born at 28 weeks of gestation is calculated below.

FIGURE 27-2 ■ Example Line of Best Fit for Gestational Age and Birth Weight

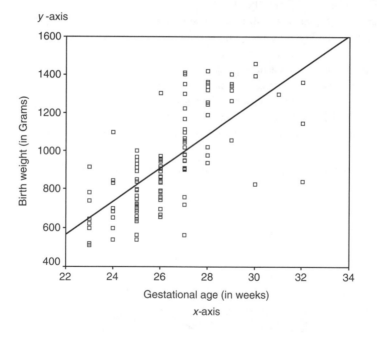

Formula: $\hat{Y} = a + bx$
In this example, $a = 500$, $b = 20$, and $x = 28$ weeks
$\hat{Y} = 500 + 20(28) = 500 + 560 = 1,060$ grams

The regression line represents $\hat{Y}$ for any given value of x. As you can see, some data points fall above the line and some fall below the line. If we substitute any x value in the regression equation and solve for y, we will obtain $\hat{Y}$ that will be somewhat different from the actual values. The distance between the $\hat{Y}$ and the actual value of y is called **residual**, and this represents the degree of error in the regression line. The regression line or the line of best fit for the data points is the unique line that will minimize error and yield the smallest residual (Burns & Grove, 2005).

■ STUDY QUESTIONS

1. What are the variables on the x- and y-axes in Figure 27-2?

2. What is the name of the type of variable represented by x and y in Figure 27-2? Is x or y the score to be predicted?

3. What is the purpose of simple linear regression analysis and the regression equation?

4. What is the point where the regression line meets the *y-axis* called? Is there more than one term for this point?

5. In $\hat{Y} = a + bx$, is a or b the slope? What does the slope represent in regression analysis?

6. Using the values $a = 500$ and $b - 20$ in Figure 27-2, what is the predicted birth weight in grams for an infant at 36 weeks of gestation?

7. Using the values $a = 500$ and $b = 20$ in Figure 27-2, what is the predicted birth weight in grams for an infant at 22 weeks of gestation?

8. Using the values $a = 500$ and $b = 20$ in Figure 27-2, what is the predicted birth weight in grams for an infant at 35 weeks of gestation?

9. Does Figure 27-2 have a positive or negative slope? Provide a rationale for your answer. Discuss the meaning of the slope of Figure 27-2.

■ ANSWERS TO STUDY QUESTIONS

1. The x variable is gestational age in weeks, and the y variable is birth weight in grams in Figure 27-2.
2. x is the independent or predictor variable. y is the dependent variable or the variable that is to be predicted by the independent variable, x.
3. Simple linear regression is conducted to estimate or predict the values of a dependent variable based on the values of an independent variable. Regression analysis is used to calculate a line of best fit based on the relationship of the independent variable x with the dependent variable y. The formula developed with regression analysis can be used to predict the dependent variable (y) values based on values of the independent variable x.
4. The point where the regression line meets the y-axis is called the y intercept and is also represented by a (see Figure 27-1). a is also called the regression constant. At the y intercept, $x = 0$.
5. b is the slope of the line of best fit (see Figure 27-1). The slope of the line indicates the amount of change in y for each one unit of change in x. b is also called the regression coefficient.
6. $\hat{Y} = a + bx$
   $\hat{Y} = 500 + 20(36) = 500 + 720 = 1{,}220$ grams
7. $\hat{Y} = a + bx$
   $\hat{Y} = 500 + 20(22) = 500 + 440 = 940$ grams
8. $\hat{Y} = a + bx$
   $\hat{Y} = 500 + 20(35) = 500 + 700 = 1{,}200$ grams
9. Figure 27-2 has a positive slope since the line extends from the lower left corner to the upper right corner and shows a positive relationship. This line shows that the increase in x (independent variable) is also associated with an increase in y (dependent variable). Thus, the independent variable gestational age is used to predict the dependent variable of birth weight. As the weeks of gestation increase, the birth weight in grams also increases, which is a positive relationship.

RESEARCH ARTICLE

Source: LeFlore, J. L., Engle, W. D., & Rosenfeld, C. (2000). Determinants of blood pressure in very low birth weight neonates: Lack of effect of antenatal steroids. *Early Human Development, 59*(1), 37–50.

Introduction

LeFlore, Engle, and Rosenfeld (2000) conducted a retrospective, cohort study (Group 1 received antenatal steroids [$n = 70$]) with matched controls (Group II did not receive antenatal steroids [$n = 46$]) to examine the effect of antenatal steroids on neonatal blood pressure (BP) in the first 72 hours of life in very low birth weight (VLBW) neonates. Additionally, the effect of other perinatal factors on BP were studied, which included estimated gestational age (EGA), birth weight (BW), and postnatal age. The results indicate that there are positive linear relationships between BP and BW, BP and EGA, and BP and postnatal age.

Relevant Study Results

BP for Group I and Group II were compared over the first 72 hours of the neonate's life. Since there were no significant differences in initial and subsequent measurements of BP between the groups, subsequent analyses were performed with the groups combined ($n = 116$). To assess the effect of BW on BP, the infants were grouped into those with BW ≤ 1,000 grams ($n = 36$) and those with BW 1,001–1,500 grams ($n = 80$). The researchers displayed the results of their analyses in figures. Figure 2 displays the relationships between postnatal age in hours and 3 BPs, systolic BP (SBP), diastolic BP (DBP), and mean BP (MBP), for infants with BW ≤ 1,000 grams. Figure 3 displays the relationship between postnatal age in hours and SBP, DBP, and MBP for infants with a BW 1,001–1,500 grams.

FIGURE 2 ■ Change in **(A)** systolic blood pressure (SBP), **(B)** diastolic blood pressure (DBP), and **(C)** mean blood pressure (MBP) in neonates ≤ 1,000 grams birth weight ($n = 36$) during the initial 72 hours postnatal. Lines represent means and 95% confidence intervals ($p < 0.0001$). Equations for lines of best fit were: SBP = 43.2 + 0.17x; DBP = 25.8 + 0.13x; MBP = 32.9 + 0.14x. In each instance, the y intercept was significantly lower ($p < 0.001$) than the value for comparable lines of best fit in infants with birth weights 1,001–1,500 grams; however, no significant differences in slopes for the lines of best fit were observed between the two birth weight groups. LeFlore, J. L., Engle, W. D., & Rosenfeld, C. (2000). Determinants of blood pressure in very low birth weight neonates: Lack of effect of antenatal steroids. *Early Human Development, 59*(1), p. 44

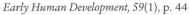

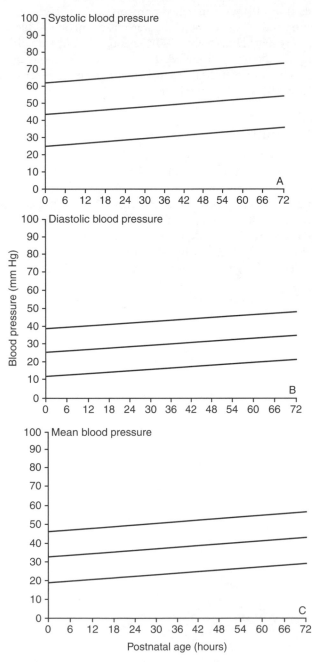

FIGURE 3 ■ Change in **(A)** systolic blood pressure (SBP), **(B)** diastolic blood pressure (DBP), and **(C)** mean blood pressure (MBP) in neonates 1,001–1,500 grams birth weight ($n = 80$) during the initial 72 hours postnatal. Lines represent means and 95% confidence intervals ($p < 0.0001$). Equations for lines of best fit were: SBP = 50.3 + 0.12x; DBP = 30.4 + 0.11x and MBP = 37.4 + 0.12x. In each instance, the y intercept was significantly greater ($p < 0.001$) than the value for comparable lines of best fit in infants with birth weight ≤1,000 grams; however, no significant differences in the slopes for the lines of best fit were observed between the two birth weight groups. LeFlore, J. L., Engle, W. D., & Rosenfeld, C. (2000). Determinants of blood pressure in very low birth weight neonates: Lack of effect of antenatal steroids. *Early Human Development, 59*(1), p. 45.

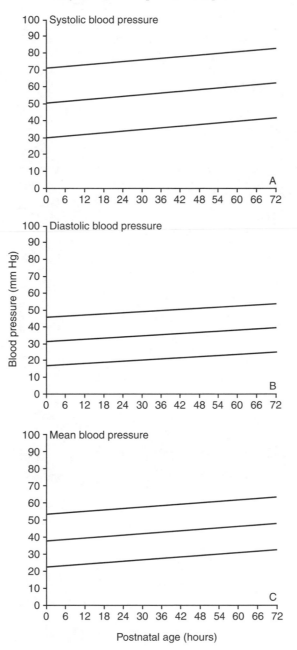

■ EXERCISE 27   Questions to be Graded

1. What are the independent and dependent variables in Figures 2, A, B, and C? How would you describe the relationship between the variables in Figures 2, A, B, and C?

2. What are the independent and dependent variables in Figures 3, A, B, and C? How would you describe the relationship between the variables in Figures 3, A, B, and C?

3. Was there a significant difference in the y intercept for the lines of best fit in Figure 2 from the y intercept for the lines of best fit in Figure 3? Provide a rationale for your answer.

4. $\hat{Y}$ represents the predicted value of y calculated using the equation $\hat{Y} = a + bx$. In Figure 2, the formula for SBP is $\hat{Y} = 43.2 + 0.17x$. Identify the y intercept and the slope in this formula. What does x represent in this formula?

5. In the legend beneath Figure 2, the authors give an equation indicating that systolic blood pressure is $SBP = 43.2 + 0.17x$. If the value of x is postnatal age of 30 hours, what is the value for $\hat{Y}$ or SBP for neonates $\leq 1,000$ grams? Show your calculations.

6. In the legend beneath Figure 2, the authors give an equation indicating that systolic blood pressure is SBP = 50.3 + 0.12x. If the value of x is postnatal age of 30 hours, what is the value for $\hat{Y}$ or SBP for neonates 1,001–1,500 grams? Show your calculations.

7. Compare the SBP readings you found in Questions 5 and 6. Explain the difference in these two readings.

8. In the legend beneath Figure 2, the authors give an equation indicating that diastolic blood pressure is DBP = 25.8 + 0.13x. If the value of x is postnatal age of 30 hours, what is the value for $\hat{Y}$ for neonates ≤ 1,000 grams? Show your calculations.

9. In the legend beneath Figure 3, the authors give an equation indicating that diastolic blood pressure is DBP = 30.4 + 0.11x. If the value of x is postnatal age of 30 hours, what is the value for $\hat{Y}$ for neonates 1,001–1,500 grams? Show your calculations.

10. In the legend beneath Figure 3, the authors give an equation indicating that diastolic blood pressure is DBP = 30.4 + 0.11x. How different is the DBP when the value of x is postnatal age of 60 hours versus the 30 hours examined in Question 9?

MULTIPLE LINEAR REGRESSION

STATISTICAL TECHNIQUE IN REVIEW

Simple linear regression was introduced in Exercise 27 and provides a means to estimate or predict the value of a dependent variable based on the value of an independent variable. **Multiple regression** is an extension of simple linear regression in which more than one independent variable is entered into the analysis to predict a dependent variable. The assumptions of multiple regression are:

1. The independent variables are measured with minimal error.
2. Variables can be treated as interval level measures.
3. The residuals are not correlated.
4. Dependent variable scores come from a normal distribution.
5. Scores are homoscedatic or equally dispersed about the line of best fit.
6. y scores have equal variance at each value of x; thus difference scores (residuals or error scores) are random and have homogenous variance (Burns & Grove, 2005).

With multiple independent variables, researchers often correlate the independent variables with the dependent variable to determine which independent variables are most highly correlated with the dependent variable. Pearson r analysis is typically used to determine correlations for interval and ratio level data. To be effective predictors, independent variables need to have strong correlations with the dependent variable but only weak correlations with the other independent variables in the equation. **Multicollinearity** occurs when the independent variables in the multiple regression equation are strongly correlated. This often happens in nursing studies, but it can be minimized by careful selection of independent variables that have limited correlation.

One of the outcomes from multiple regression analysis is an R^2 value. For the addition of each independent variable to the regression formula, the change in R^2 is reported. The R^2 is used to calculate the percentage of variance that is predicted by the regression formula. For example, the independent variables of number of cigarettes smoked, systolic blood pressure (SBP), and body mass index (BMI) were used to predict the incidence of myocardial infarction (MI) in older adults. The $R^2 = 0.387$ and the percent of variance predicted is calculated by $R^2 \times 100\%$. In this example, the % of variance predicted by the regression formula is calculated by $0.387 \times 100\% = 38.7\%$. This means that 38.7% of the variance in the incidence of MI in the older adult is predicted by the independent variables of number of cigarettes smoked, SBP, and BMI. The significance of an R^2 value is tested with an analysis of variance (ANOVA) (see Exercises 36 and/or 37). The statistic for ANOVA is F, and a significant F value indicates that the regression equation has significantly predicted the variation in the dependent variable and that the R^2 value is not a random variation.

RESEARCH ARTICLE

Source: Zalon, M. L. (2004). Correlates of recovery among older adults after major abdominal surgery. *Nursing Research, 53*(2), 99–106.

Introduction

Zalon (2004) conducted a predictive correlational study to determine whether the independent variables of pain, depression, and fatigue were predictive of older adults' return to functional status and self-perception of recovery after abdominal surgery. The study involved adults who were 60 years of age or older who had undergone major abdominal surgery. "Data were collected during hospitalization ($n = 192$), then 3–5 days ($n = 141$), 1 month ($n = 132$), and 3 months after discharge to home ($n = 126$) using the Brief Pain Inventory, the Geriatric Depression Scale-Short Form, the Modified Fatigue Symptom Checklist, the Enforced Social Dependence Scale, and the Self-Perception of Recovery Scale" (Zalon, 2004, p. 99). The conclusions of the study were that pain, depression, and fatigue are predictive of the functional status and self-perception of recovery in older adults following surgery. Interventions are needed to reduce pain, depression, and fatigue to improve the postoperative recovery of older adults.

Research Study Results

Zalon (2004) conducted Pearson r correlations among the independent variables pain, depression, and fatigue, and with the dependent variables functional status and self-perception of recovery. These variables were correlated at hospitalization, 3–5 days post-discharge, 1 month post-discharge, and 3 months post-discharge, and the correlation values are presented in Table 2. It is assumed that alpha was set at 0.05 for this study.

TABLE 2 ■ Correlation Matrix for Study Variables at Each Time Interval					
	1	2	3	4	5
Initial (Hospitalization)					
1. Pain	–	.37**	.52**	–	−.20**
2. Depression		–	.53**	–	−.09
3. Fatigue			–	–	−.20**
4. Functional status				–	–
5. Self-perception of recovery					–
3–5 Days post-discharge					
1. Pain	–	.27**	.39**	.12	−.25**
2. Depression		–	.60**	.36**	−.28**
3. Fatigue			–	.26**	−.13
4. Functional status				–	−.09
5. Self-perception of recovery					–
One Month post-discharge					
1. Pain	–	.33**	.22**	.33**	−.44**
2. Depression		–	.51**	.50**	−.50**
3. Fatigue			–	.42**	−.32**
4. Functional status				–	−.50**
5. Self-perceptional of recovery					–
Three Months Post-Discharge					
1. Pain	–	.26**	.50**	.39**	−.24**
2. Depression		–	.54**	.43**	−.35**
3. Fatigue			–	.46**	−.34**
4. Functional status				–	−.53**
5. Self-perception of recovery					–

**P < .01.
Zalon, M.L. (2004). Correlates of recovery among older adults after major abdominal surgery. *Nursing Research, 53*(2), p. 104.

Multiple regression analysis was conducted to determine if pain, depression, and fatigue were predictive of functional status and self-perception of recovery. The results of the multiple regression analysis indicated that pain, depression, and fatigue are significantly predictive of the patient's self-perception of recovery and functional status. "Pain, depression, and fatigue explained 13.4% of the variation in functional status at 3 to 5 days, 30.8% at 1 month, and 29.1% at 3 months after discharge. These three factors also explain 5.6% of the variation in self-perception of recovery during hospitalization, 12.3% at 3 to 5 days, 33.2% at 1 month, and 16.1% at 3 months after discharge. . . . Pain, depression, and fatigue are important factors to consider in the provision of care to abdominal surgery patients with a relatively uncomplicated postoperative course. Specific interventions to reduce pain, depression, and fatigue need to be evaluated for their impact on the postoperative recovery of older adults" (Zalon, 2004, p. 99) (see Table 3).

TABLE 3 ■ Regression of Pain, Fatigue, and Depression on Functional Status and Self-Perception of Recovery

n		169	137	131	126
Dependent variable	Independent variables	Initial B	3–5 Days B	1 Month B	3 Months B
Functional status					
	Pain		.001	.06*	.05*
	Depression		.85**	.84***	.44**
	Fatigue		.04	.13*	.09*
F			6.94***	18.82***	16.69***
R^2			.134	.308	.291
Self-perception of recovery					
	Pain	−.15	−.22*	−.35	.08
	Depression	.79	−3.23*	−3.01*	−1.31*
	Fatigue	−.25	.31	−.13	−.22
F		3.28*	6.24**	21.06***	7.83***
R^2		.056	.123	.332	.161

*$p < .05$. **$p < .01$. ***$p < .001$.
Zalon, M.L. (2004). Correlates of recovery among older adults after major abdominal surgery. *Nursing Research, 53*(2), p. 104.

■ STUDY QUESTIONS

1. What is the purpose of multiple regression analysis?

2. What were the independent and dependent variables in this study?

3. Why did Zalon (2004) correlate the independent and dependent variables with each other? What results would provide the strongest study outcomes for regression analysis?

4. Which independent variable was most highly correlated with functional status at 3–5 days post-discharge? Provide a rationale for your answer.

5. Were the independent variables pain, depression, and fatigue significantly correlated with functional status at 3–5 days post-discharge? Provide a rationale for your answer.

6. Were the independent variables pain, depression, and fatigue significantly correlated with each other at 3–5 days post-discharge? How does this affect the multiple regression results?

7. What was the multiple regression result for functional status at 3–5 days post-discharge? Was this result significant? Provide a rationale for your answer.

8. Did the regression results indicate that pain, depression, and fatigue provided a greater prediction of functional status at 1 month after discharge or at 3–5 days post-discharge? Provide a rationale for your answer.

9. What was the percentage of variance explained by the regression analysis for functional status at 3 months? Provide your calculations.

10. Discuss the multiple regression analysis results for functional status. What do these results indicate for practice?

ANSWERS TO STUDY QUESTIONS

1. Multiple regression analysis is conducted to predict an outcome or dependent variable using two or more independent variables. This analysis is an extension of simple linear regression where more than one independent variable is entered into the analysis to develop a formula for predicting the dependent variable.

2. In the Zalon (2004) study, there were three independent variables: pain, depression, and fatigue. These three independent variables were used to predict the dependent variables functional status and self-perception of recovery in an elderly population.

3. With multiple independent variables, researchers often correlate the independent variables with each other and with the dependent variable. Pearson r analysis is usually used to determine correlations for interval and ratio level data. To be effective predictors, independent variables need to have strong correlations with the dependent variable but only weak correlations with the other independent variables in the equation.

4. The independent variable depression was most highly correlated with the dependent variable functional status with an $r = .36^{**}$ at 3–5 days post-discharge. Pain had a correlation of $r = .12$ with functional status, and fatigue was correlated at $r = .26^{**}$ with functional status. The farther the r value is from the zero (0) and the closer it is to +1 or –1, the stronger the correlation.

5. The independent variables depression and fatigue were significantly correlated with the dependent variable functional status with $r = .36^{**}$ and $r = .26^{**}$, respectively. The ** indicate that $p < .01$ for these r values, which are significant since the p values are less than alpha that was set at 0.05. Pain had a correlation of $r = .12$ with functional status, which was not significant since it did not have an * (see Table 3).

6. The three independent variables were significantly correlated with each other at 3–5 days post-discharge as indicated by the r values with **. Pain was significantly correlated with depression at $r = .27^{**}$, pain was significantly correlated with fatigue at $r = .39^{**}$, and depression was significantly correlated with fatigue at $r = .60^{**}$ (see Table 3). Independent variables are stronger predictors of a dependent variable if they are not strongly correlated with each other. Since pain, fatigue, and depression were significantly correlated with each other, this probably resulted in a smaller R^2 value and percentage of variance explained for functional status than would have been obtained had the independent variables had limited correlation with each other.

7. The multiple regression result was $R^2 = .134$ for functional status 3–5 days post-discharge. The analysis of variance (ANOVA) was conducted to determine the significance of the results and the results were significant with $F = 6.94^{***}$, $p < .001$. This result was significant as indicated by the *** and the p value < 0.05 or alpha.

8. Multiple regression results indicated a stronger prediction of functional status at 1 month after discharge with $R^2 = .308$ than at 3–5 days post-discharge with $R^2 = .134$. The larger R^2 value indicates that pain, depression, and fatigue predicted a greater amount of variance in functional status at 1 month after discharge than 3–5 days. The results were also more significant at 1 month post-discharge with $F = 18.82^{***}$, $p < .001$ than the results at 3–5 post-discharge at $F = 6.94^{***}$, $p < .001$. The larger the F value, the more significant the results when there is comparable sample size, but the actual p value is needed for the results to know just how much more significant $F = 18.82$ is than $F = 6.94$.

9. 29.1% variance was explained for functional status at 3 months after discharge.
$$\% \text{ variance} = R^2 \times 100\% = 0.291 \times 100\% = 29.1\%$$

10. The multiple regression results were significant at 3–5 days, 1 month, and 3 months post-discharge as indicated by $F = 6.94^{***}$, $F = 18.82^{***}$, and $F = 16.69^{***}$, respectively. These results indicate that pain, depression, and fatigue were predictive of functional status in this study. The clinical implications for this study are that older patients need effective management of their pain, depression, and fatigue following abdominal surgery to promote their return to functional status. Zalon (2004) stressed the importance of identifying specific interventions to reduce pain, depression, and fatigue to promote postoperative recovery in older adults. Additional research is need to determine if these findings are reflected in other samples.

■ EXERCISE 28   Questions to be Graded

1. Was multiple regression analysis the appropriate analysis technique to conduct in this study? Provide a rationale for your answer.

2. Which independent variable had the strongest correlation with self-perception of recovery at 1 month after discharge? Provide a rationale for your answer.

3. Were the independent variables pain, depression, and fatigue significantly correlated with self-perception of recovery at 1 month after discharge? Provide a rationale for your answer.

4. Did multicollinearity occur in this study? Provide a rationale for your answer.

5. Did the regression results indicate that pain, depression, and fatigue provided a greater prediction of self-perception of recovery at 1 month after discharge, or at 3–5 days post-discharge? Provide a rationale for your answer.

6. What was the percentage of variance explained by the regression analysis for self-perception of recovery at 1 month after discharge? Provide your calculations.

7. What was the percentage of variance explained by the regression analysis for functional status at 1 month after discharge? Provide your calculations.

8. Was the percentage of variance explained for self-perception of recovery lower than the percentage of variance explained for functional status at 1 month after discharge? Discuss the meaning of these results.

9. Discuss the multiple regression analysis results for self-perception of recovery following discharge. What do these results indicate for practice?

10. Are these results ready to be generalized to older adults after other types of surgery, such as joint replacement? Provide a rationale for your answer.

29 *t*-TEST FOR INDEPENDENT GROUPS I

STATISTICAL TECHNIQUE IN REVIEW

The **t-test** is a parametric analysis technique used to determine significant differences between the scores obtained from two groups. The *t*-test uses the standard deviation to estimate the standard error of the sampling distribution and examines the differences between the means of the two groups. Since the *t*-test is considered fairly easy to calculate, researchers often use it in determining differences between two groups. When interpreting the results of *t*-tests, the larger the calculated *t* ratio, in absolute value, the greater the difference between the two groups. The significance of a *t* ratio can be determined by comparison with the critical values in a statistical table for the *t* distribution using the degrees of freedom (*df*) for the study. The formula for *df* for an independent *t*-test is:

$$df = \text{number of subjects in sample 1} + \text{number of subjects in sample 2} - 2$$

The *t*-test can only be used once to examine data from two study samples, otherwise the Type 1 error rate (alpha) may be inflated. A Type I error occurs when the researcher rejects the null hypothesis when it is in actuality true. Thus if researchers run multiple *t*-tests to evaluate differences of various aspects of a study's data, this is considered a misuse of the *t*-test and often leads to an increased risk for a Type I error or finding two groups significantly different when they are not. To correct for the risk of a Type I error, the researcher can perform a Bonferroni procedure. The Bonferroni procedure is a simple calculation in which the alpha is divided by the number of *t*-tests run on different aspects of the study data. The resulting number is used as the alpha or level of significance for each of the *t*-tests conducted. For example, if a study's alpha was set at 0.05 and the researcher planned on conducting 5 *t*-tests on the study data, the alpha would be divided by the 5 *t*-tests (0.05 ÷ 5 = 0.01), with a resulting alpha of 0.01 to be used to determine significant differences in the study. The Bonferroni procedure formula is:

Alpha (α) ÷ number of *t*-tests performed on study data = more stringent study α to determine the significance of study results.

The *t*-test for independent groups includes the following assumptions:

1. The raw scores in the population are normally distributed.
2. The dependent variable(s) is (are) measured at the interval or ratio levels.
3. The two groups examined for differences have equal variance, which is best achieved by a random sample and random assignment to groups.
4. All observations within each group are independent.

The *t*-test is robust, meaning the results are reliable even if one of the assumptions has been violated. However, the *t*-test is not robust regarding between-samples or within-samples independence assumptions, or with respect to extreme violation of the assumption of normality. Sample groups do not need to be of equal sizes but rather of equal variance. Groups are independent if the two sets of data were not taken from the same subjects and if the scores are not related. Thus, paired or matched groups are dependent, not independent; but a randomly selected sample with random assignment to groups does produce independent groups (Burns & Grove, 2005).

RESEARCH ARTICLE

Source: Kristofferzon, M., Löfmark, R., & Carlsson, M. (2005). Perceived coping, social support, and quality of life 1 month after myocardial infarction: A comparison between Swedish women and men. *Heart & Lung, 34*(1), 39–50.

Introduction

Kristofferzon, Löfmark, and Carlsson (2005) conducted a comparative-descriptive study to determine if women and men differ in their perceived coping, social support, and quality of life one month post myocardial infarction (MI). The sample of convenience included 171 subjects, 74 women and 97 men. Each participant completed a study-specific questionnaire (demographics and risk factors), the JCS-60 (measured use of coping strategies), the social network and social support questionnaire (measured social participation and emotional support), the SF-36 Health Survey (measured perceived health-related quality of life), and the QLI (measured perceived quality of life). In addition, the researchers conducted a chart review of each participant's medical record. In this study the results showed that "compared with men, women used more evasive and supportive coping and rated psychologic aspects of the heart disease as more problematic to manage. More women perceived available support from friends and grandchildren, and more men perceived available support from their partner. Women rated lower levels in physical and psychologic dimensions of quality of life" (Kristofferzon et al., 2005, p. 39).

Relevant Study Results

"A consecutive series of patients was selected from the medical records in 1 hospital between August 1999 and July 2001 for women and between August 1999 and August 2000 for men. With regard to a lower incidence rate of MI in women, a longer selection period was needed for them. . . . We decided to include 100 women and 100 men to have a comfortable margin for dropouts.

"An introductory letter, informed consent form, and questionnaires were mailed to eligible subjects 1 month after an acute MI. After 1 week, the first author phoned the patients. Those interested in participating returned the signed consent form and the completed questionnaires to the investigator within 1 to 2 weeks. The same questionnaires were mailed to the subjects on 3 occasions, 1, 4, and 12 months after MI. Data from 1 month are presented in this article" (Kristofferzon et al., 2005, p. 41).

"Of the target population of 338 women, 20% died before inclusion, 35% did not meet the inclusion criteria, and 23% declined participation; of the target population of 317 men, the corresponding numbers were 17%, 27%, and 26%, respectively. . . . The final sample consisted of 74 women and 97 men" (Kristofferzon et al., 2005, p. 41).

In Table VI, are the quality of life measures reported by Kristofferzon et al. (2005) in their study of women and men following an MI. The level of significance or alpha for this study was set at 0.05.

TABLE VI ■ Quality of Life Experienced by Women and Men (N = 171)				
INSTRUMENTS AND COMPONENTS/SCALES	WOMEN (n = 74) MEAN (SD)	MEN (n = 97) MEAN (SD)	T VALUE (DF = 169)	P VALUE
SF-36 (0 = low QoL, 100 = high QoL)				
The Physical Component Score (PCS)*	48.5 (5.7)	51.1 (7.4)	−2.50	0.01
The Mental Component Score (MCS)†	48.2 (7.6)	51.4 (7.5)	−2.74	0.007
Physical Functioning (PF)	51.3 (23.7)	58.6 (24.1)	−1.98	0.049
Role-Physical (RP)	4.7 (14.1)	12.6 (23.7)	−2.54‡	0.007
Bodily Pain (BP)	57.6 (26.2)	62.5 (27.3)		0.24
General Health (GH)	51.1 (17.6)	54.2 (20.1)		0.30
Vitality (VT)	39.8 (19.0)	47.5 (23.2)	−2.31§	0.02
Social Functioning (SF)	61.0 (27.4)	66.1 (23.2)		0.19
Role-Emotional (RE)	27.5 (39.5)	37.8 (42.7)		0.11
Mental Health (MH)	62.3 (22.9)	72.7 (20.1)	−3.15	0.002
QLI (0 = low QoL, 30 = high QoL)				
Total Scale	20.1 (3.5)	21.2 (3.6)	−2.06	0.04
Health Functioning	17.9 (4.1)	19.3 (4.6)	−1.99	0.049
Socioeconomic	22.6 (3.6)	22.9 (3.7)		0.58
Psychologic/spiritual	19.6 (4.6)	21.1 (4.3)	−2.10	0.04
Family (N = 69 women and 94 men)	25.6 (4.7)	26.0 (3.9)		0.51

*PCS = PF, RP, BP, GH. †MCS = VT, SF, RE, MH. ‡df = 161. §df = 168. QoL = Quality of life; QLI, Quality-of-Life Index-Cardiac Version.
Kristofferzon, M., Löfmark, R., & Carlsson, M. (2005). Perceived coping, social support, and quality of life 1 month after myocardial infarction: A comparison between Swedish women and men. *Heart & Lung, 34*(1), p. 47.

■ STUDY QUESTIONS

1. *t* = −1.99 describes the difference between women and men post myocardial infarction (MI) for what variable?

2. Consider *t* = −2.74 and *t* = −2.31. Which calculated *t* ratio has the smaller *p* value? Provide a rationale for your answer.

3. Examine the results in Table VI. Which *t* ratio listed in the table had the largest *p* value? What was the focus of this *t*-test, and were the results significant? Provide a rationale for your answer.

4. What is *df*? Why is it important to know the *df* for a *t* ratio? How would you calculate the *df* for a *t*-test, and what is the *df* for this study?

5. What is the cause of an increased risk for Type I errors when *t*-tests are conducted? How might researchers eliminate the increased risk for a Type I error in a study?

6. Given the information presented in Table VI, calculate a Bonferroni procedure for this study.

7. Does this study meet the assumptions for the *t*-test? Provide a rationale for your answer.

8. What sampling method did the researchers use in this study? Provide a rationale for your answer.

9. What level of data is analyzed by means and standard deviations? Is this level of data compatible with the assumptions for the *t*-test? Provide a rationale for your answer.

10. Is the sample size adequate to detect significant differences between the two groups in this study?

■ ANSWERS TO STUDY QUESTIONS

1. $t = -1.99$ describes the difference in health functioning between women and men after a MI.

2. $t = -2.74$, $p = 0.007$; $t = -2.31$, $p = 0.02$. $t = -2.74$ has the smaller p value at $p = 0.007$ than $t = -2.31$ with $p = 0.02$. The smaller p value indicates more significant findings.

3. Both $t = -1.98$ (physical functioning) and $t = -1.99$ (health functioning) had equal and the largest p values at $p = 0.049$ that were still considered statistically significant. These two t ratios indicated the differences between males and females for physical functioning and health functioning in this sample. These t values are significant because the $p = 0.049$ value is smaller than alpha (α) that was set at 0.05 for this study.

4. $df =$ degrees of freedom. Degrees of freedom (df) is a mathematical equation that describes the freedom of a particular score's value to vary based on the other existing scores' values and the sum of the scores (Burns & Grove, 2005). The df for an analysis technique allows you to look up t ratios on a statistical table that includes t distributions to determine their significance. The df calculations vary based on the analysis technique conducted. Thus, the formula for df for the t-test for independent groups is:

   $df =$ number in group 1 + number in group 2 − 2

   For this study $df =$ 74 women + 97 men − 2 = 169

5. The conduct of multiple t-tests causes an increased risk for Type I errors. If only one t-test is performed on study data, the risk of Type I error does not increase. A Bonferroni procedure reduces the risk for Type I errors.

6. The Bonferroni procedure is calculated by alpha ÷ number of t-tests conducted on study data. For this study only 9 t values are provided in Table VI, but the p values indicate that 15 t-tests were conducted and only 9 of these were significant. Thus, the Bonferroni calculation includes:

   0.05 (alpha) ÷ 15 (number of t-tests conducted in a study) = 0.0033 (Bonferroni result)

7. Answers may vary. Yes, the study meets the required assumptions for the t-test. The researchers do not indicate if the scores from the two groups are normally distributed, so it is assumed that they are. The study variables are measured at least at the interval level as indicated by the measurement methods used in the study. The researchers mentioned the longer length of time required to recruit an adequate number of women to ensure a more equal variance between the groups. However, the variance of scores would have been ensured more if the original sample had been randomly selected. The two groups were independent since they were formed based on gender (male and female) with no intent to match subjects on any variable.

8. A nonprobability, convenience sampling method was used in the study. The researchers recruited consecutive patients from one hospital over a period of time, which is consistent with a convenience sampling method. If a random sampling method had been used to obtain the sample, the researcher would have indicated this in the sample section of the study.

9. Means and standard deviations are calculated for variables that are measured at the interval and ratio levels. These analysis techniques are used to describe study variables. The t-test is a parametric analysis technique to detect differences between two groups. The dependent variables in a study must be measured at the interval or ratio levels in order for a t-test to be conducted (see the assumptions for the t-test).

10. Answers may vary. The sample size is adequate since 9 t values were significant in this study. If significant differences are detected, then the sample size is adequate. However, if you use the Bonferroni procedure, there is only one t value ($t = -3.15$, $p = 0.002$) that is significant at the 0.0033 level of significance identified in Question 6. Thus, the sample size might be viewed as too small since only one t value is significant. Or one might conclude that the differences between the males and females post MI are not significant.

■ **EXERCISE 29**   Questions to be Graded

1. Were the groups in this study independent or dependent? Provide a rationale for your answer.

2. $t = -3.15$ describes the difference between women and men for what variable in this study? Is this value significant? Provide a rationale for your answer.

3. Is $t = -1.99$ significant? Provide a rationale for your answer. Discuss the meaning of this result in this study.

4. Examine the t ratios in Table VI. Which t ratio indicates the largest difference between the males and females post MI in this study? Is this t ratio significant? Provide a rationale for your answer.

5. Consider $t = -2.50$ and $t = -2.54$. Which t ratio has the smaller p value? Provide a rationale for your answer. What does this result mean?

6. What is a Type I error? Is there a risk of a Type I error in this study? Provide a rationale for your answer.

7. Should a Bonferroni procedure be conducted in this study? Provide a rationale for your answer.

8. If researchers conducted 9 *t*-tests on their study data. What alpha level should be used to determine significant differences between the two groups in the study? Provide your calculations.

9. The authors reported multiple *df* values in Table VI. Why were different *df* values reported for this study?

10. What does the *t* value for the Physical Component Score tell you about men and women post MI? If this result was consistent with previous research, how might you use this knowledge in your practice?

30

t-TEST FOR INDEPENDENT GROUPS II

STATISTICAL TECHNIQUE IN REVIEW

One of the most common parametric analysis techniques used to test for differences between statistical measures (namely means) of two groups is the t-test. The t-test for independent groups can be conducted to examine differences between two independent or unrelated groups that are often formed by the random assignment of subjects to the treatment and comparison groups. Groups are also independent if they are selected from two different settings, two different points in time, or are not matched in any way. The t-test yields a p value, which indicates the probability of assuming that the null hypothesis is true. A difference between two groups is said to be significant when p is equal or less than alpha (α), which is often set at $\alpha = 0.05$. When two groups are significantly different for a study variable, the null hypothesis is rejected.

Exercise 29 provides a detailed discussion of the t-test for independent groups, and you might review this information. Remember that a t-test can only be conducted once when analyzing the study data without an inflation of the Type I error rate. To correct for the escalating risk of the Type I error, the researcher can perform a Bonferroni procedure. The Bonferroni procedure is a simple calculation in which the study alpha is divided by the number of t-tests conducted on the study's data. The resulting value is a more stringent alpha level for determining the significance of the t-tests conducted for the study.

RESEARCH ARTICLE

 Source: Tel, H., & Tel, H. (2006). The effect of individualized education on the transfer anxiety of patients with myocardial infarction and their families. *Heart & Lung, 35*(2), 101-7.

Introduction

Tel and Tel (2006) conducted a study "to determine the effect of individualized education on the anxiety level of patients with myocardial infarction [MI] and their families who are being transferred from the coronary care unit (CCU) to the general care unit. . . . The study consisted of experimental and comparison groups, and took place in a CCU of a teaching hospital. The study included 90 patients with myocardial infarction who were admitted to the CCU and 90 individuals who were the relatives of the patients. . . . Patients in the CCU and their relatives experience anxiety. An individualized education program is effective in decreasing the anxiety of patients and their relatives when the patients are transferred from the CCU to the general care unit" (Tel & Tel, 2006, p. 101).

Relevant Study Results

Tel and Tel (2006) conducted their quasi-experimental study in a university hospital setting. "Ninety patients with a first-time diagnosis of MI in the CCU who were conscious and could communicate, and who agreed to participate in the study, and 90 of their relatives who were the patients' spouse or child and had primary responsibility for their care were accepted into the study. Forty-five patients and their 45 relatives were in the experimental group, and 45 patients and their 45 relatives were in the comparison group. . . . Data were collected in the study using a personal characteristics information form, a disease information form [to measure information level], and the Spielberger State-Trait Anxiety Inventory (STAI) [to measure anxiety level]. . . . To prevent interaction between groups that might affect the study outcome, data were first collected from the comparison group" and then the experimental group (Tel & Tel, 2006, pp. 102–3).

The demographic characteristics of the two groups were compared with chi-square and an "independent-sample, *t*-test was used for the comparison between the experimental and comparison groups' information and anxiety scores" (Tel & Tel, 2006, p. 103). Initial *t*-test analyses indicated that there were no differences in the baseline anxiety and informational scores for the patients and their relatives at the start of the study ($p > 0.05$ with $\alpha = 0.05$). Following the implementation of the individualized educational program, the results indicated a statistically significant difference between the anxiety scores for the two groups of patients ($t = 3.875, p < 0.001$) and relatives ($p < 0.01$). The experimental group's informational scores were significantly different for patients ($t = 16.819, p < 0.001$) and relatives ($t = 35.174, p < 0.001$).

"In this study, it was seen that individualized education was effective in decreasing the anxiety period of patients and their relatives. Individualized education was also found to have an effect on the transfer anxiety of patients and their relatives, resulting in a decrease in the patients' level of anxiety at transfer and preventing the relatives' anxiety level from increasing. The information scores of patients and their relatives after education in the experimental group were significantly higher than those of the comparison group, which shows that this development was related to the education that was individualized and based on specific needs" (Tel & Tel, pp. 105–6). The findings from this study were consistent with other studies, so the researchers made the following recommendations for practice: "(1) Patients should be evaluated emotionally on admission to the CCU and at routine intervals, and (2) an individualized educational program focused on meeting the needs of patients and their relatives, and a CCU transfer policy should be developed" (Tel & Tel, 2006, p. 106).

■ STUDY QUESTIONS

1. What were the independent and dependent variables in this study?

2. The researchers conducted multiple *t*-tests in determining the results for this study. What might be the effect of these *t*-tests on study results?

3. Should the researchers have conducted a Bonferroni procedure as part of their data analysis? Provide a rationale for your answer.

4. If Tel and Tel (2006) conducted 5 *t*-tests during their data analysis, what should their level of significance become using the Bonferroni procedure if originally $\alpha = 0.05$? Provide your calculations.

5. The experimental group's informational scores were significantly different for patients ($t = 16.819$, $p < 0.001$). With the Bonferroni procedure calculated in Question 4, is this result statistically significant? Provide a rationale for your answer.

6. The experimental group's informational scores were significantly different for patients ($t = 16.819$, $p < 0.001$). What do these results mean?

7. For the result in Question 6, should the null hypothesis be accepted or rejected? Provide a rationale for your answer.

8. How many subjects participated in this study? Describe the number of subjects in each group.

9. What were the numbers and types of subjects in the experimental and comparison groups, and were these study strengths or weaknesses? Provide a rationale for your answer.

10. What were the sample criteria for this study? Were these sample criteria strengths or weaknesses? Provide a rationale for your answer.

ANSWERS TO STUDY QUESTIONS

1. The independent variable or treatment was the individualized educational program. The two dependent or outcome variables were information and anxiety levels.

2. The *t*-test can only be used once in examining the data from a study without inflating the risk for a Type I error or saying something is significant when it is not. To correct for the increased risk of a Type I error, the researchers needed to perform a Bonferroni procedure.

3. Yes, the researchers would have strengthened their study results if they had used the Bonferroni procedure in determining the significant differences between the experimental and comparison groups. Since several *t*-tests were conducted on the study data, the Bonferroni procedure would have reduced the risk of a Type I error of saying the two groups were different when they were not.

4. The Bonferroni procedure is a simple calculation in which the study alpha level is divided by the number of *t*-tests conducted in the study. The more stringent alpha level that results is used to determine significant differences between the experimental and comparison groups.

Calculation: Bonferroni procedure = α ÷ number *t*-tests = more stringent alpha
Bonferroni procedure = $0.05 \div 5 = 0.01$

Thus, any *t*-test results with $p \leq 0.01$ would be considered significant if the Bonferroni procedure was used to determine the significance of the results.

5. Yes, this result is statistically significant with the Bonferroni procedure since the result was significant at $p < 0.001$ and with the Bonferroni procedure the more stringent $\alpha = 0.01$. The *p* value < 0.001 is smaller than $\alpha = 0.01$, making the results significant.

6. The experimental group's informational scores were statistically significantly different for patients ($t = 16.819$, $p < 0.001$). This result means that the patients in the experimental group who got the individualized educational program had significantly different informational scores than the patients in the comparison groups. This result supports the effectiveness of the intervention, an individualized educational program, to improve the patients' informational scores.

7. Based on the results presented in Question 6, the null hypothesis is rejected. The null hypothesis states: There is no difference in the informational scores of patients who received an individualized education program versus those who do not. Since the results were significant at $p < 0.001$, the null hypothesis is rejected because a significant difference does exist between the two groups on informational scores.

8. A total of 180 subjects participated in this study. Ninety subjects (45 MI patients and their 45 relatives) were in the experimental group, and 90 subjects (45 MI patients and their 45 relatives) were in the comparison group.

9. The experimental and comparison groups each had 90 subjects. In addition, each group had an equal number of MI patients (45) and relatives (45). The equal group sizes and the equal distribution of MI patients and their relatives in each group are study strengths. Since the groups are the same size and have the same distribution of MI patients and their relatives, this reduces the potential for sampling error in the study results.

10. The sample criteria for the patients in this study were: patients with a first-time diagnosis of MI in the CCU, who were conscious, could communicate, and agreed to participate in the study. The sample criteria for the relatives in this study were: relatives were the patients' spouse or child and had primary responsibility for the MI patients' care. These sample criteria limited the patients to those with first MI who were conscious and could communicate, which reduced the number of extraneous variables that might have affected the study outcomes. They also ensured that the relatives had a close rapport with the MI patients since they were primarily responsible for their care.

■ EXERCISE 30   Questions to be Graded

1. What were the two groups in this study? Were these groups independent or dependent? Provide a rationale for your answer.

2. Was an independent *t*-test the appropriate analysis technique for this study? Provide a rationale for your answer.

3. The baseline anxiety and information scores were not significantly different between the experimental and comparison groups. What does this mean? Does this strengthen or weaken the results of the study? Provide a rationale for your answer.

4. If Tel and Tel (2006) had conducted 7 *t*-tests during their data analyses, what would their alpha be using the Bonferroni procedure if the initial study $\alpha = 0.05$? Provide your calculations.

5. The results indicated a statistically significant difference between the anxiety scores for the two groups of patients ($t = 3.875, p < 0.001$). What do these results mean?

6. For the result in Question 5, should the null hypothesis be accepted or rejected? Provide a rationale for your answer.

7. The results indicated a statistically significant difference between the anxiety scores for the two groups of patients ($t = 3.875, p < 0.001$). Are these results also significant at the 0.01 level? Provide a rationale for your answer.

8. What variables were measured in this study? What measurement methods were used to measure these variables?

9. In the Relevant Study Results from the Tel and Tel (2006) study, what strengthened the findings from this study? Does this increase the ability to generalize the study findings to other populations?

10. How might you use these study findings in practice?

31

t-TEST FOR DEPENDENT GROUPS

STATISTICAL TECHNIQUE IN REVIEW

The **_t_-test for dependent groups** is a parametric analysis technique used to determine statistical differences between two related samples or groups. Groups are dependent or related because they were matched as part of the design to ensure similarities between the two groups and thus reduce the effect of extraneous variables. For example, two groups might be matched on gender so an equal number of males and females are in each group, thus reducing the extraneous effect of gender on the study results. The researcher's decision to match groups is determined by the study being conducted and is detailed in the study design. In previous research, groups have most commonly been matched for age, gender, ethnicity, diagnoses, and status of illness. Matching the groups strengthens the study design by reducing the effect of extraneous variables controlled by matching. Groups are also dependent when scores used in the analysis are obtained from the same subjects under different conditions, such as pretest and posttest study design. In this type of design, a single group of subjects is exposed to pretest, treatment, and posttest. Subjects are referred to as serving as their own control during the pretest that is then compared with the posttest scores following the treatment. This is a weak quasi-experimental design since it is difficult to determine the effects of a treatment without comparison to a separate control group. The assumptions for the *t*-test for dependent groups are:

1. The distribution of scores is normal or approximately normally distributed.
2. The dependent variable(s) is (are) measured at interval or ratio levels.
3. The groups examined for differences are dependent based on matching or subjects serving as their own control.
4. The differences between the paired scores are independent (Burns & Grove, 2005).

RESEARCH ARTICLE

Source: Kim, C., Junes, K., & Song, R. (2003). Effects of a health-promotion program on cardiovascular risk factors, health behaviors, and life satisfaction in institutionalized elderly women. *International Journal of Nursing Studies, 40*(4), 375–81.

Introduction

Kim, Junes, and Song (2003) conducted a quasi-experimental study with a one group pretest-posttest design. "A convenient sample of 21 elderly women was recruited from a home for elderly people." (Kim et al., 2000, p. 376). The purpose of the study was to determine the health benefits of a 3-month health-promotion program for institutionalized elderly women on cardiovascular risk factors, health behaviors, and life satisfaction. These researchers found the following positive effects from the program: reductions in total risk score, improved health behaviors, and improved life satisfaction. However, Kim et al. (2003) noted a decrease in these positive effects 3 months after the completion of the health-promotion program.

Relevant Study Results

A total of 25 women were enrolled in the health-promotion program and 21 subjects completed the program with three sets of outcome assessments at pretest, 3 months, and 6 months. The mean age of the subjects was 77 years, and 90% of them had been diagnosed with one or more chronic diseases. The significance level of the study was set at $\alpha = 0.05$. The results from the study are presented in the two tables that follow. Table 2 describes the health-promotion program's effects on cardiovascular risk factors, and Table 3 describes the effects on health behaviors. The third dependent variable of this study was life satisfaction, which was significantly improved from pretest to the end of the health-promotion program at 3 months and at 6 months follow-up.

TABLE 2 ■ Program Effects on Cardiovascular Risk Factors

	PRETEST	3 MONTHS		6 MONTHS	
Variable	M (SD)	M (SD)	Paired t^a	M (SD)	Paired t^b
Total risk score	20.1 (4.5)	16.8 (3.2)	4.14*	18.1 (4.0)	2.56*
Cholesterol	200.2 (29.1)	189.6 (25.3)	2.03*	192.7 (22.1)	1.73
Triglyceride	164.2 (42.0)	150.4 (44.1)	2.58*	142.9 (53.5)	2.20*
BMI	22.7 (3.0)	22.1 (3.0)	3.44*	22.9 (3.0)	−0.80
Systolic BP	121.7 (14.6)	117.2 (12.3)	1.57	115.6 (13.4)	1.66

BMI (body mass index), *BP* (blood pressure)
*$p < 0.05$.
[a] Paired *t*-test results between the pretest and 3-month measures.
[b] Paired *t*-test results between the pretest and 6-month measures.
Kim, C., Junes, K., & Song, R. (2003). Effects of a health-promotion program on cardiovascular risk factors, health behaviors, and life satisfaction in institutionalized elderly women. *International Journal of Nursing Studies, 40*(4), p. 378.

TABLE 3 ■ Program Effects on Health Behaviour

	PRETEST	3 MONTHS		6 MONTHS	
Variable	M (SD)	M (SD)	Paired t^a	M (SD)	Paired t^b
Total health behavior	66.3 (8.1)	69.7 (5.0)	−3.02*	68.1 (5.1)	−1.34
Health responsibility	2.19 (0.5)	2.13 (0.3)	1.03	2.29 (0.3)	−1.39
Exercise	1.88 (0.3)	2.58 (0.3)	−7.75*	2.29 (0.4)	−3.93*
Diet behavior	3.41 (0.3)	3.47 (0.2)	−0.93	3.26 (0.3)	2.00
Stress management	2.39 (0.4)	2.44 (0.3)	−0.65	2.45 (0.3)	−0.70
Smoking behavior	2.85 (0.8)	2.92 (0.8)	−1.45	3.01 (0.7)	−0.96

*$p < 0.05$.
[a] Paired *t*-test results between the pretest and 3-month measures.
[b] Paired *t*-test results between the pretest and 6-month measures.
Kim, C., Junes, K., & Song, R. (2003). Effects of a health-promotion program on cardiovascular risk factors, health behaviors, and life satisfaction in institutionalized elderly women. *International Journal of Nursing Studies, 40*(4), p. 379.

■ STUDY QUESTIONS

1. What clues do you have that this study had "dependent groups?"

2. Which *t* ratio or value in Table 3 is the greatest for the 6-month follow-up? Which variable is being examined for differences between the pretest and 6-month follow-up by this *t* ratio?

3. Which *t* ratio or value listed in Table 2 is the smallest in determining the difference between the pretest and 6-month follow-up? This *t* ratio was calculated to determine the change in which variable from pretest to 6 months after the intervention?

4. $t = -0.93$ is the result for what variable in this study? Is this *t* ratio significant? Provide a rationale for your answer.

5. Compare the pretest to 3 months and 6 months *t* ratios for BMI from Table 2. What is your conclusion regarding the effects of the health-promotion intervention on the BMI long term?

6. The *t*-test for dependent groups is conducted in research for what purpose?

7. What is the smallest, significant *t* ratio listed in Table 3? Provide a rationale for your answer.

8. Why do you think that the smaller *t* ratios are not statistically significant?

9. How would you describe the result *t* = –1.45 in this study?

ANSWERS TO STUDY QUESTIONS

1. This study was conducted using a *one group* pretest-posttest design in which the subjects serve as their own control. The subjects' outcomes at 3 and 6 months were compared with their pretest values. The single sample pretest-posttest design indicates that the groups were dependent or related. In Tables 2 and 3 the *t*-tests are identified as paired *t*-tests, which are conducted on dependent groups.

2. *t* = –3.93 (Exercise) is the largest *t* ratio at 6 months, as listed in Table 3.

3. *t* = –0.80 (BMI) represents the smallest *t*-ratio at 6 months, as listed in Table 2.

4. *t* = –0.93 indicates the difference in Diet behavior from pretest to 3 months. This *t*-ratio does not have an asterisk (*) next to it in Table 3; therefore, it is not statistically significant. The asterisk directs the reader to the footnotes at the bottom of the table where the asterisk is said to represent $p < 0.05$, the least stringent acceptable value for statistical significance.

5. *t* = 3.44* (3 months) and *t* = –0.80 (6 months). At 3 months, the difference in BMI (body mass index) from pretest was statistically significant with *t* = 3.44*, $p < 0.05$. At 6 months, the difference in BMI from pretest was no longer statistically significant with *t* = –0.80. These results indicate that although initially the BMI decreased significantly from the pretest (mean = 22.7) to 3 months (mean = 22.1), the BMI actually increased at 6 months (mean = 22.9). Thus, the health-promotion intervention did not have a positive long-term effect on the subject's BMI, since the subjects demonstrated an increase in BMI versus a decrease.

6. The *t*-test for dependent groups is conducted to determine statistical differences between two related or dependent groups. The *t*-test can be used to determine differences between two dependent groups following a treatment and also for comparing and contrasting two groups for a selected variable. Paired *t*-test is another name for the *t*-test for dependent groups.

7. *t* = –3.02*, $p < 0.05$ is the smallest significant *t* ratio listed in Table 3. The –3.02 is the smallest *t* ratio with an *, indicating that Total health behavior was statistically significant from pretest to 3 months in this study at $p < 0.05$.

8. The small *t* ratios indicate small relative differences between the two groups that are usually not statistically significantly different, especially in small sample studies. The larger the calculated *t* ratios, the smaller the observed *p* values and the more likely one will reject the null hypothesis, since the groups are significantly different.

9. The result *t* = –1.45 indicates that there is no statistically significant difference in Smoking behavior from pretest to 3 months in this sample. Thus, the null hypothesis would be accepted, which states the health-promotion intervention did not have an effect on Smoking behavior.

■ EXERCISE 31   Questions to be Graded

1. What are the two groups whose results are reflected by the *t* ratios in Tables 2 and 3?

2. Which *t* ratio in Table 2 represents the greatest relative or standardized difference between the pretest and 3 months outcomes? Is this *t* ratio statistically significant? Provide a rationale for your answer.

3. Which *t* ratio listed in Table 3 represents the smallest relative difference between the pretest and 3 months? Is this *t* ratio statistically significant? What does this result mean?

4. What are the assumptions for conducting a *t*-test for dependent groups in a study? Which of these assumptions do you think were met by this study?

5. Compare the 3 months and 6 months *t* ratios for the variable Exercise from Table 3. What is your conclusion about the long-term effect of the health-promotion intervention on Exercise in this study?

6. What is the smallest, significant *t* ratio listed in Table 2? Provide a rationale for your answer.

7. Why are the larger *t* ratios more likely to be statistically significant?

8. Did the health-promotion program have a statistically significant effect on Systolic blood pressure (BP) in this study? Provide a rationale for your answer.

9. Examine the means and standard deviations for Systolic BP at pretest, 3 months (completion of the treatment), and 6 months. What do these results indicate? Are these results clinically important? Provide a rationale for your answer.

10. Is this study design strong or weak? Provide a rationale for your answer.

◼ BONUS QUESTION

Would you, as a health care provider, implement this intervention at your facility based on the Total Risk Score results? Provide a rationale for your answer.

SIGNIFICANCE OF CORRELATION COEFFICIENT

STATISTICAL TECHNIQUE IN REVIEW

The **significance of a correlation coefficient** is determined by a mathematical calculation that determines whether the correlations or relationships found in a study apply to the population from which the sample was obtained. In other words, the calculation of significance determines if the correlation is significantly different from zero, or no correlation (Burns & Grove, 2005). If you have any questions about correlation coefficients, please see Exercises 23 and 24.

The significance of a correlation coefficient can be determined by the calculation of a t value. The significance of the t value calculated can be determined using the table of critical t values and degrees of freedom (df) equal to $n - 2$ found in most research textbooks (Burns & Grove, 2005). The formula for calculating t is as follows:

$$t = \frac{r\sqrt{n-2}}{\sqrt{1-r^2}}$$

r = Pearson's product-moment correlation coefficient
n = sample size of paired scores
$df = n - 2$
Example: $r = 0.76$, $n = 15$

$$t = \frac{0.76\sqrt{15-2}}{\sqrt{1-(0.76^2)}} = \frac{2.74}{\sqrt{0.422}} = \frac{2.74}{0.65} = 4.22$$

The significance of the correlation coefficient is important to determine along with the strength and direction (positive or negative) of the relationship. Correlation coefficients that you might assume are significant because they are moderate or large may not be because of the small size of the sample. If a study has a small sample, a larger correlation coefficient is needed to detect statistically significant relationships. In addition, one might assume that some small correlation coefficients are insignificant but in fact they are significant with large samples. The t values and their corresponding p values can also be determined as part of the computer analysis of correlational data to identify statistically significant relationships.

RESEARCH ARTICLE

Source: O'Mahony, S., Goulet, J., Kornblith, A., Abbatiello, G., Clarke, B., Kless-Siegel, S., Breitbart, W., & Payne, R. (2005). Desire for hastened death, cancer pain, and depression: Report of a longitudinal observational study. *Journal of Pain and Symptom Management, 29*(5), 446–57.

Introduction

O'Mahony et al. (2005) conducted an observational study of patients receiving antineoplastic and supportive treatments to understand the effect of cancer pain on a desire for hastened death. The sample of 64 cancer patients were each interviewed at baseline and 4 weeks after the treatments. The investigators compiled the subjects' responses regarding pain, symptoms of depression, perceived social support, spiritual well-being, significant medical events, satisfaction with analgesic regimen, and opioid side effects. The researchers found that an improvement in depression, which means the patients were less depressed, was significantly associated or correlated with an improvement in the desire for hastened death, which means their desire for hastened death was decreased. Also, significant correlations were found between desire for hastened death and the variables of cancer pain severity, degree of interference with physical functioning, perceived lack of social support, and low levels of physical functioning.

Relevant Study Results

O'Mahony et al. (2005) presented their correlational coefficients in Table 3, which includes the relationships between the baseline desire for hastened death and the baseline measurements of the other study variables. The study level of significance or alpha (α) was set at 0.05. The p values in Table 3 are the probabilities identified for the correlational values obtained in this study. If the p value is less than $\alpha = 0.05$, then the results are statistically significant. The smaller the p value, the more significant the results.

TABLE 3 ■ Correlation of Baseline Desire for Hastened Death with Baseline Measures

Baseline Variables	Pearson Correlation	p
Age	0.11	0.41
BDI-II (Depression)	0.43	< 0.01
BPI (Pain)	0.27	0.03
FACT (Spiritual Well-Being)	−0.38	< 0.01
STAI (Anxiety)	0.28	0.03
Bottomley (Social Support)	0.38	< 0.01
KPRS (Physical Functioning)	−0.40	< 0.01

O'Mahony, S., Goulet, J., Kornblith, A., Abbatiello, G., Clarke, B., Kless-Siegel, S., Breitbart, W., & Payne, R. (2005). Desire for hastened death, cancer pain, and depression: Report of a longitudinal observational study. Reprinted from the *Journal of Pain and Symptom Management, 29*(5):446-47, with permission from copyright © 2005, The U.S. Cancer Pain Relief Committee.

■ STUDY QUESTIONS

1. $r = -0.38$ represents the relationship between which two variables?

2. Describe the relationship for $r = -0.38$. Be sure to include the direction, strength, and statistical significance of this relationship.

3. Is $r = -0.38$ clinically important? Provide a rationale for your answer.

4. Calculate the degrees of freedom (*df*) for this study.

5. Calculate the *t* value associated with $r = -0.38$.

6. Using the results from Question 5, determine the statistical significance of $r = -0.38$. Describe that significance.

7. How would you incorporate the knowledge about the relationship between spiritual well-being and desire for hastened death into your clinical practice, since this relationship is statistically significant and clinically important?

8. Calculate the *t* value for $r = 0.11$.

9. Is $r = 0.11$ statistically significant? Provide a rationale for your answer.

ANSWERS TO STUDY QUESTIONS

1. $r = -0.38$ represents the relationship between the FACT scale, which measures spiritual well-being, and desire for hastened death. The values for these variables were obtained at baseline or at the start of the study.

2. $r = -0.38$ is a moderate, negative, statistically significant relationship between spiritual well-being and desire for hastened death. This means that as spiritual well-being increases, desire for hastened death decreases. The relationship is negative as indicated by the minus (–) sign and of moderate strength since it is > -0.3 and < -0.5. The $r = -0.38$ is statistically significant as indicated by $p < 0.01$, which is less than $\alpha = 0.05$.

3. Clinical importance is determined by examining the percentage of variance explained between the two variables of spiritual well-being and desire for hastened death, which is 14% in this study. This value indicates that 14% of the variance in hastened death is determined by spiritual well-being, which is clinically important since it is >10% (see Exercise 24).

$$\text{Percentage of variance explained} = r^2 \times 100\% = (-0.38)^2 \times 100\% = 0.144 \times 100\% = 14\%$$

4. $df = 62$

$$df = n - 2 \qquad df = 64 - 2 \qquad df = 62$$

5. $t = -3.22$

$$t = \frac{-0.38\sqrt{64-2}}{\sqrt{1-(-0.38)^2}} = \frac{-2.99}{\sqrt{0.86}} = \frac{-2.99}{0.93} = -3.22$$

6. In this study, the researchers indicated that for $r = -0.38$, $p < 0.01$. Look at a table of critical t values for a two-tailed t-test in your textbook, and you should find that $t = -3.22$ and $df = 62$ is statistically significant at least at $p < 0.01$. The absolute critical t value $= 2.65$, $\alpha = 0.01$; therefore, the $t = -3.22$ is statistically significant since it is greater than the tabled value. Thus, $r = -0.38$ is statistically significant as indicated in the article and also by calculating the t value and determining its statistical significance in a table of critical t values.

7. $r = -0.38$ is both clinically important (14% variance explained) and statistically significant ($p < 0.01$). Realizing that the relationship between spiritual well-being and desire for hastened death is a significant, moderate, negative relationship with 14% of the variance explained, the health care provider caring for cancer patients can include assessment and support of spiritual well-being into the plan of care to decrease the desire for hastened death. If spiritual well-being is promoted from the onset, a health care provider can assist a patient in coping with his or her cancer. However, this is an area that does need additional research with a variety of cancer patients to strengthen the knowledge for use in practice.

8. $t = 0.88$

$$t = \frac{0.11\sqrt{64-2}}{\sqrt{1-(0.11)^2}} = \frac{0.87}{\sqrt{0.99}} = \frac{0.87}{0.99} = 0.879 = 0.88$$

9. No, $r = 0.11$ is not statistically significant. For this study, $p = 0.41$ was found for $r = 0.11$ in Table 3. A similar p value can be found in the t distribution table in your research textbook for $t = 0.88$ and $df = 62$.

■ EXERCISE 32   Questions to be Graded

1. $r = 0.43$ represents the relationship between which two variables?

2. Describe the relationship for $r = 0.43$. Be sure to include the direction (positive or negative) and strength of the relationship in your discussion.

3. Calculate the t value associated with $r = 0.43$.

4. Calculate the degrees of freedom (df) for a study that has 80 subjects, which is needed to calculate the significance of the correlation coefficients for the study.

5. Is $r = 0.43$ statistically significant? Discuss how you have arrived at your answer.

6. Is $r = 0.43$ clinically important? Provide a rationale for your answer.

7. How would you incorporate the knowledge about the $r = 0.43$ results into your clinical practice?

8. Calculate the t value for $r = 0.27$.

9. Is $r = 0.27$ clinically important? Is $r = 0.27$ statistically significant?

10. Would you use the knowledge about the relationship between pain and desire for hastened death in your clinical practice? Provide a rationale for your answer.

STANDARD ERROR OF THE MEAN: 95TH CONFIDENCE INTERVAL

STATISTICAL TECHNIQUE IN REVIEW

The standard error of the mean (SE_M) represents the error to be expected when the mean from a smaller sample of the population is used to calculate the standard deviation of the population mean. The SE_M allows for error in the sample and can be calculated at the 95th and 99th levels. When stated as the 95% confidence interval (CI), the researchers are saying that there is a 95% chance that the mean is correct or a 5% chance that the mean is an error. The interval is represented by two numbers, with the true mean falling somewhere in between the two values. In order to calculate the CI, the SE_M is multiplied by 1.96. This number is then added to and subtracted from the mean; the result is the range or the 95th CI. The formulas for calculating the SE_M and the 95th CI are:

Formula for SE_M

$$SE_M = \frac{SD}{\sqrt{N}}$$

Formula for 95th CI

$$\text{95th CI} = \text{Mean} \pm 1.96\, SE_M$$

For example, if $N = 100$, $SD = 15$, and mean = 54, the SE_M is 1.50.
95th CI = $54 \pm 1.96(1.50) = 54 - 2.94 = 51.06$ and $54 + 2.94 = 56.94$.
95% of the time the true mean is between 51.06 and 56.94 and CI is expressed as (51.06, 56.94).

RESEARCH ARTICLE

Source: Westman, E. C., Yancy, W. S., Edman, J. S. Tomlin, K. F., & Perkins, C. E. (2002). Effect of 6-month adherence to a very low carbohydrate diet program. *The American Journal of Medicine, 113*(1), 30–6.

Introduction

Westman et al. (2002) conducted an uncontrolled study using 51 overweight healthy volunteers to determine the effects of a 6-month low-carbohydrate diet on weight loss and metabolic function. They recruited persons who wanted to lose weight and screened them with a medical history and physical examination, which included laboratory testing, urinary ketone measurements, and an electrocardiogram. The researchers concluded that "a very low carbohydrate diet program led to sustained weight loss during a 6-month period" (Westman et al., 2002, p. 30). "Limitations of this study include the uncontrolled design, self-report of several variables, and the use of skin-fold calipers to estimate fat mass. Because only healthy volunteers were studied, caution should be used when generalizing these results to patients with medical illnesses. Although the dropout rate and adherence to this diet program are similar to that seen in other weight loss studies, the possibility of adverse effects in those who did not adhere to the program cannot be eliminated. . . . Further controlled research is needed to estimate the risks and benefits of this diet in healthy persons and in patients with other medical conditions" (Westman et al., 2002. p. 35).

Relevant Study Results

The subjects were placed on a < 25g/d carbohydrate diet until 40% of the subject's self-determined weight reduction goal was met. At that point the carbohydrate requirement was raised to 50g/d. The subjects were encouraged to exercise at least 20 minutes 3 times a week, and to drink at least six 8-ounce glasses of water a day. They were also provided with a multivitamin formula, essential oil formula, diet formula, and chromium picolinate supplements. During the 6 months, the participants also attended group meetings every other week for the first 12 weeks, followed by every month for 3 months. During the meetings, the subjects self-reported what they were eating, and received instruction on low-carbohydrate diets. Repeat lab testing was administered throughout the length of the study.

The subjects overall body weight was reduced by 10.3% ± 5.9% during the study, with a mean decrease in body mass index of $3.2 \pm 1.9 \text{ kg/m}^2$. The adverse effects of the diet were reported as constipation for 68% of the participants, bad breath for 63%, headaches for 51%, hair loss for 10%, and increases in menstrual bleeding for 3% of the women. Table 2 shows the effects of the diet program on metabolic indices, and Table 3 shows the effects on serum lipid levels and 24-hour urinary excretion.

TABLE 2 ■ Effect of Very Low Carbohydrate Diet Program on Metabolic Indices

Parameter	Baseline ($n = 41$)	Week 8 ($n = 41$)	Week 16 ($n = 38$)	Week 24 ($n = 41$)	Change from Baseline to Week 24 Mean Difference (95% Confidence Interval)	P value
	Mean ± SD					
Sodium (mmol/L)	142 ± 1	141 ± 2	140 ± 2	139 ± 1	−3 (−4 to −2)	<0.001
Chloride (mmol/L)	104 ± 2	104 ± 2	104 ± 3	103 ± 2	−1 (−2 to 0)	0.02
Bicarbonate (mmol/L)	27 ± 2	26 ± 2	24 ± 2	25 ± 2	−2 (−3 to −1)	<0.001
Uric acid (mg/dL)	5.3 ± 1	5.2 ± 1	5.2 ± 1	5.0 ± 1	−0.3 (−1 to 0)	0.01
Asparlate aminotransferase (U/L)	26 ± 9	23 ± 8	23 ± 9	22 ± 9	−4 (−6 to −2)	0.002
Total bilirubin (mg/dL)	0.7 ± 0.3	0.6 ± 0.2	0.7 ± 0.2	0.8 ± 0.3	0.1 (0 to 0.2)	<0.001
Alkaline phosphatase (U/L)	75 ± 20	66 ± 14	65 ± 14	69 ± 15	−6 (−11 to −1)	0.02
Blood urea nitrogen (mg/dL)	13 ± 3	15 ± 5	16 ± 5	15 ± 5	2 (1 to 3)	<0.001
Creatinine (mg/dL)	0.9 ± 0.2	0.9 ± 0.2	0.8 ± 0.2	0.8 ± 0.2	−0.1 (−0.13 to 0)	0.06
Blood urea nitrogen/creatinine ratio	15 ± 5	18 ± 5	20 ± 5	19 ± 5.5	4 (3.8 to 4.1)	<0.001

TABLE 3 ■ Effect of Very Low Carbohydrate Diet Program on Serum Lipid Level and 24-Hour Urinary Excretion

Parameter	Baseline (n = 41)	Week 8 (n = 41)	Week 16 (n = 38)	Week 24 (n = 41)	Change from Baseline to Week 24 Mean Difference (95% Confidence Interval)	P value
	Mean ± SD					
Total cholesterol (mg/dL)	214 ± 35	201 ± 37	201 ± 42	203 ± 36	−11 (−19 to −3)	0.006
LDL cholesterol (mg/dL)	136 ± 32	136 ± 36	128 ± 39	126 ± 34	−10 (−13 to −2)	0.01
HDL cholesterol (mg/dL)	52 ± 14	49 ± 11	58 ± 13	62 ± 15	10 (8 to 12)	<0.001
Non-HDL cholesterol (mg/dL)	162 ± 37	152 ± 39	143 ± 42	141 ± 37	−21 (−29 to −13)	<0.001
Triglycerides (mg/dL)	130 ± 62	82 ± 32	75 ± 30	74 ± 33	−56 (−70 to −42)	<0.001
Total cholesterol/HDL cholesterol ratio	4.3 ± 1.3	4.3 ± 1.2	3.6 ± 1.0	3.4 ± 0.9	−0.9 (−1.1 to −0.7)	<0.001
Triglycerides/HDL cholesterol ratio	2.8 ± 2.0	1.8 ± 1.0	1.4 ± 0.7	1.3 ± 0.9	−1.5 (−1.9 to −1.1)	<0.001
Urinary creatinine clearance (mL/min)*	124 ± 30	126 ± 33	128 ± 38	129 ± 26	5 (−4 to 16)	0.33
Urinary calcium (mg/24 h)*	162 ± 109	289 ± 152	306 ± 159	248 ± 120	86 (44 to 128)	<0.001
Urinary uric acid (mg/24 h)*	540 ± 202	630 ± 337	542 ± 240	635 ± 155	95 (20 to 170)	0.02
Urinary protein (mg/24 h)*	119 ± 54	145 ± 85	130 ± 53	134 ± 50	15 (−10 to 40)	0.25

*Urinary changes are assessed using a paired test comparing baseline to week 24; n=24 as each time point.
HDL = high density lipoprotein; LDL = Low density lipoprotein; non-HDL cholesterol = total cholesterol minus HDL cholesterol.
Westman, E. C., Yancy, W. S., Edman, J. S., Tomlin, K. F., & Perkins, C. E. (2002). Effect of 6-month adherence to a very low carbohydrate diet program. *The American Journal of Medicine, 113*(1), p. 34. Copyright © 2002, with permission from Excerpta Medica, Inc.

■ STUDY QUESTIONS

1. What is the mean difference from baseline to week 24 for Uric Acid?

2. Between what two numbers does the true mean for blood urea nitrogen (BUN) lie 95% of the time, which is the 95% confidence interval (CI)?

3. In Table 2, which parameter or variable has the largest mean difference from baseline to week 24?

4. In Table 3, which parameter or variable has the largest confidence interval (CI)?

5. In a study, the sample size was $N = 130$, $SD = 5$, and the mean $= 50$. Calculate the SE_M and the 95th CI for this study.

6. How is the non-HDL cholesterol calculated?

7. During the initial part of this study, the subjects were not restricted in the amount of protein that they consumed, but the total cholesterol was reduced at the end of the study. Provide a rationale for this finding.

8. This study lasted only 6 months. In examining Table 2, can you see any potential long-term side effects from this diet?

9. In Tables 2 and 3, the n value for week 16 was 38 or $n = 38$ but was $n = 41$ at baseline, week 8, and week 24. Why was the sample size less at week 16 as compared to the other measurement points?

10. Is the very low-carbohydrate diet healthy? Provide a rationale for your answer.

ANSWERS TO STUDY QUESTIONS

1. The answer is –0.3, which can be found in Table 2 in the column Change from Baseline to Week 24. This figure can also be calculated by taking the mean at 24 weeks minus the mean at baseline or 5.0 – 5.3 = –0.3.

2. The true mean for BUN is somewhere between 1 and 3. This answer is found in Table 2 and is the 95th CI for BUN.

3. Alkaline phosphatase at –6 has the largest difference from baseline to week 24 of the parameters listed in Table 2.

4. Urinary uric acid has the largest CI that ranges from 20 to 170 in Table 33-2.

5. Use the formula for the 95th CI presented at the beginning of this exercise.

$$SE_M = 5 \div \sqrt{130} = 5 \div 11.40 = 0.439 = 0.44$$
$$95\text{th CI} = \text{Mean} \pm 1.96\ SE_M, \ 1.96 \times 0.44 = 0.862 = 0.86$$
$$50 - 0.86 = 49.14 \text{ and } 50 + 0.86 = 50.86$$
$$95\text{th CI is } (49.14, 50.86).$$

6. At the bottom of Table 3, the non-HDL cholesterol = total cholesterol – HDL cholesterol.

7. Other studies where weight loss has occurred have resulted in a decrease in the total cholesterol levels and a reduction in both LDL and triglyceride levels. This is usually the result of weight loss as well as the diet consumed. Low carbohydrate intake leads to the use of fats and proteins to fuel the body, which results in a decrease in LDL, total cholesterol, and triglycerides.

8. Continuing the low-carbohydrate diet could possibly result in decreases in the bicarbonate level and increases in the urinary excretion of calcium and uric acid. High-protein diets can also be problematic to those who have decreased kidney functions and can result in increased BUN and creatinine levels. Low-carbohydrate diets are often associated with an increased consumption of fat that can result in gallbladder disease.

9. The *n* represents the number of subjects who participated in the testing at the different times (baseline, week 8, week 16, and week 24). During week 16, only 38 subjects participated in getting their lab drawn, and 41 subjects participated at the other testing times.

10. The use of very low-carbohydrate diets is controversial. People have lost weight on this type of diet as they did in this study. Potential adverse effects noted by the researchers include calcium oxalate and urate kidney stone, vomiting, amenorrhea, hypercholesterolemia, and water-soluble vitamin deficiencies. It should also be noted that this was an uncontrolled study with self-reporting of food preferences, so the accuracy of the study results could be in question based on the accuracy of the subjects' reported data. The researchers provided the subjects with nutritional supplements, which further confuse the long-term effects of the low-carbohydrate diets.

■ EXERCISE 33   Questions to be Graded

1. What is the mean difference from baseline to week 24 for total cholesterol?

2. What is the mean difference from baseline to week 24 for bicarbonate?

3. Between what two numbers does the true mean for triglycerides exist 95% of the time, which is the 95% confidence interval (CI)?

4. Between what two numbers does the true mean for creatinine exist 95% of the time, which is the 95% confidence interval (CI)?

5. Did the HDL cholesterol value change significantly from baseline to week 24? Is this result clinically significant?

6. In a study, the sample size was $N = 150$, $SD = 9$, and the mean = 48. Calculate the SE_M and the 95th confidence interval for this study.

7. In Table 2, which parameter or variable has the smallest confidence interval?

8. The Atkins Center provided funding and training for the research staff. Would this have an effect on the outcomes of this study? Provide a rationale for your answer.

9. In this study, 51 subjects were enrolled, but only 41 completed it. Identify some possible reasons for the sample mortality of 10 subjects.

10. This was an uncontrolled study. Identify ways to improve the control of the study and thus strengthen the study design.

34

STANDARD ERROR OF THE MEAN: 99TH CONFIDENCE INTERVAL

STATISTICAL TECHNIQUE IN REVIEW

The standard error of the mean (SE_M) represents the error to be expected when the mean from a smaller sample of the population is used to calculate the standard deviation of the population mean. This allows for error in the sample and can be calculated at the 95th or 99th confidence intervals (CI). Researchers might identify the 99th CI or the 99% CI when presenting their study results, and these CIs are really expressing the same idea. When stated as 99% CI, the researchers are saying that there is a 99% chance that the mean is within the confidence interval and a 1% chance of error. The CI is represented by two numbers with the true mean falling somewhere in between those two numbers. In order to calculate the standard error of the mean, you need the number of subjects and the standard deviation (SD). Take the SD and divide it by the square root of the number of subjects and the result is the SE_M. In order to calculate the 99th CI, the SE_M is multiplied by 2.58. This number is then added and subtracted from the study mean; the result is the range of the 99th CI:

Formula for SE_M

$$SE_M = \frac{SD}{\sqrt{N}}$$

Formula for 99th CI

$$99\text{th CI} = \text{Mean} \pm 2.58\ SE_M$$

An example of such a calculation is: $N = 100$, $SD = 15$, and mean = 54.
$SE_M = 15 \div 10 = 1.5$. The 99th CI = 54 ±1.5(2.58) = 54 − 3.87 = 50.13 and 54 + 3.87 = 57.87. The true mean is between 50.13 and 57.87 or the 99th CI = (50.13, 57.87).

RESEARCH ARTICLE

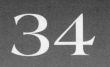 **Source:** Galiè, N., Hinderliter, A. L., Torbicki, A., Fourme, T., Simonneau, G., Pulido, T. et al. (2003). Effects of the oral endothelin-receptor antagonist bosentan on echocardiographic and doppler measures in patients with pulmonary arterial hypertension. *Journal of the American College of Cardiology, 41*(8), 1380–6.

Introduction

Galiè et al. (2003) conducted a double-blind, randomized, placebo-controlled trial to investigate the effects of bosentan on several echocardiographic and doppler variables in patients with pulmonary arterial hypertension. The study was made up of 85 subjects who were enrolled in the BREATHE-1 (Bosentan Randomized trial for Endothelin Antagonist Therapy for pulmonary hypotension) study. The treatment group mean difference after 16 weeks of treatment with bosentan was an increase of 37 meters in the 6-minute walk.

Relevant Study Results

"Bosentan is an endothelin-receptor antagonist that inhibits endothelin, a chemical messenger released by cells that line the inside of the blood vessels, and causes narrowing of the blood vessels. Administration of bosentan leads to a decrease in the symptoms of pulmonary hypertension, such as exercise intolerance. For this study, two different doses of the drug were implemented to determine the efficacy of the drug at different levels. Twenty-nine subjects received a placebo and 56 received bosentan 125 mg or 250 mg twice daily. Six-minute walk tests and echocardiograms were performed at baseline and after 16 weeks of treatment." (Galiè et al., 2003, p. 1380).

The researchers found that bosentan improved the distance walked in 6 minutes with a mean difference between treatment groups of 37 meters. "Bosentan improves RV [right ventricular] systolic function and LV [left ventricular] early diastolic filling and leads to a decrease in RV dilation and an increase in LV size in patients with PAH [pulmonary arterial hypotension], which results in an increase in cardiac index and an improvement in cardiac function" (Galiè et al., 2003, p. 1380). The treatment group had a smaller percentage of reduction in RV enlargement and an increase in the LV dimensions, which suggests that the drug plays a part in delaying the effects of pulmonary hypertension on the heart. This led the researchers to state that the use of bosentan therapy "favorably influences parameters that predict survival in patients with PAH" (Galiè et al., 2003, p. 1386). The echocardiographic and Doppler variables that were analyzed and the baseline data for the study groups are recorded in Tables 2 and 3.

TABLE 2 ■ Baseline Echocardiographic Variables of Patients by Treatment Group								
	PLACEBO		BOSENTAN GROUPS COMBINED		125 mg OF BOSENTAN		250 mg OF BOSENTAN	
Variables	n	Mean ± SD	n	Mean ± SD	n	Mean ± SD	n	Mean ± SD
RV end-diastolic area, cm^2	24	27 ±8	44	30 ± 11	21	32 ± 11	23	28 ± 11
RV end-systolic area, cm^2	24	22 ±8	42	25 ± 10	21	26 ± 10	21	24 ±9
RV percent change in area, %	24	18 ±11	42	18 ± 11	21	21 ± 13	21	15 ±8
LV end-diastolic area, cm^2	19	16 ±7	37	14 ± 6	18	13 ± 5	19	16 ±6
LV end-systolic area, cm^2	18	11 ±6	37	10 ± 4	18	9 ± 4	19	11 ±5
LV systolic eccentricity index	27	1.86 ± 1.35	52	1.65 ± 0.38	27	1.67 ± 0.37	25	1.64 ± 0.40
LV diastolic eccentricity index	28	1.82 ± 1.03	52	1.75 ± 0.45	27	1.83 ± 0.47	25	1.66 ± 0.43
RV:LV diastolic areas ratio	19	2.22 ± 1.54	37	2.44 ± 1.48	18	2.84 ± 1.39	19	2.06 ± 1.50
IVC minimum diameter, cm	19	1.29 ± 0.54	42	1.45 ± 0.54	23	1.51 ± 0.62	19	1.38 ± 0.43
Pericardial effusion score, %*	29	45*	56	45*	29	48*	27	41*

* % of patients with any degree of pericardial effusion.
IVC = inferior vena cava; LV = left ventricle; RV = right ventricle.
Galiè, N., et al. (2003). Effects of the oral endothelin-receptor antagonist bosentan on echocardiographic and doppler measures in patients with pulmonary arterial hypertension. Reprinted from *The Journal of the American College of Cardiology,* 41(8):1380-1386, copyright © 2003, with permission from The American College of Cardiology Foundation.

TABLE 3 ■ Baseline Echocardiographic Variables of Patients by Treatment Group

Variables	n	PLACEBO Mean ± SD	n	BOSENTAN GROUPS COMBINED Mean ± SD	n	125 mg OF BOSENTAN Mean ± SD	n	250 mg OF BOSENTAN Mean ± SD
RV acceleration time, ms	27	76 ± 21	50	75 ± 24	25	78 ± 30	25	72 ± 17
RV ejection time, ms	27	283 ± 40	50	291 ± 42	25	298 ± 39	25	283 ± 44
Doppler RV index	26	0.50 ± 0.24	45	0.54 ± 0.19	22	0.50 ± 0.17	23	0.58 ± 0.21
Maximal TV regurgitant velocity, cm/s	25	438 ± 70	46	427 ± 57	23	431 ± 54	23	423 ± 60
LV stroke volume, ml	26	50 ± 19	55	52 ± 18	28	49 ± 17	27	55 ± 18
Heart rate, beats/min	27	86 ± 14	55	81 ± 13	28	80 ± 12	27	82 ± 14
Cardiac index, 1/min/m²	26	2.51 ± 0.90	55	2.47 ± 0.83	28	2.31 ± 0.69	27	2.64 ± 0.94
Doppler MV peak E velocity, cm/s	24	49 ± 16	53	53 ± 20	27	54 ± 22	26	52 ± 19
Doppler MV E/A ratio	24	0.73 ± 0.25	53	0.81 ± 0.33	27	0.82 ± 0.39	26	0.80 ± 0.25
Doppler MV time-velocity integral, cm	24	12.3 ± 2.7	53	13.0 ± 4.0	27	13.2 ± 4.3	26	12.75 ± 3.7

LV = left ventricle; MV = mitral valve; RV = right ventricle; TV = tricuspid valve.
Galiè, N. et al. (2003). Effects of the oral endothelin-receptor antagonist bosentan on echocardiographic and doppler measures in patients with pulmonary arterial hypertension. Reprinted from *The Journal of the American College of Cardiology, 41*(8):1380-1386, copyright © 2003, with permission from The American College of Cardiology Foundation.

■ STUDY QUESTIONS

1. What are the mean and standard deviation for LV systolic eccentricity index in the placebo group?

2. What are the mean and standard deviation for IVC minimum diameter (cm) in the 125 mg of bosentan group?

3. Using the formula provided in the "Statistical Technique in Review" section, calculate the SE_M for the RV: LV diastolic areas ratio for the 125 mg bosentan group. Round your answer to two decimal places.

4. Using the formula provided in the "Statistical Technique in Review" section, calculate the SE_M for the IVC minimum diameter (cm) for the 250 mg bosentan group. Round your answer to two decimal places.

5. Using your answer from Question 3, calculate the 99th confidence interval (CI) for the RV:LV diastolic areas ratio for the 125 mg bosentan group. Round your answer to two decimal places.

6. This study is described as a double-blind, randomized, placebo-controlled trial. What do those terms mean?

7. Write a null hypothesis for this study.

8. Tables 2 and 3 show the changes in the variables from baseline to after the treatment. Some of the changes are negative numbers. Provide a rationale for the negative numbers.

9. Use your answer from Question 4 and calculate the 99th confidence interval (CI) for the IVC minimum diameter (cm) for the 250 mg bosentan group. Round your answer to two decimal places.

■ ANSWERS TO STUDY QUESTIONS

1. The mean is 1.86, and the standard deviation is 1.35 for the LV systolic eccentricity index in the placebo group (see Table 2).
2. The mean is 1.51, and the standard deviation is 0.62 for the IVC minimum diameter (cm) in the 125 mg of bosentan group (see Table 2).
3. The information needed for the calculation is found in Table 2. $N = 18$ and standard deviation = 1.39. 1.39 divided by square root of 18 or 4.24 = 0.3278. Rounding this answer to two decimal places is .33, as in the following calculations:

$$SE_M = \frac{1.39}{\sqrt{18}} = \frac{1.39}{4.24} = 0.3278 = 0.33$$

4. The information needed for the calculation is found in Table 2. $N = 19$ and standard deviation = 0.43. 0.43 divided by square root of 19 or 4.36 = 0.099. The answer rounded to two decimal places is 0.10, as in the following calculations:

$$SE_M = \frac{0.43}{\sqrt{19}} = \frac{0.43}{4.36} = 0.099 = 0.10$$

5. The SE_M for RV:LV diastolic areas ratio for the 125mg bosentan group is 0.33. In order to calculate the 99th CI, you first multiply the SE_M by 2.58 ($.33 \times 2.58 = 0.851 = 0.85$), then add and subtract that answer from the mean 2.84. The 99th CI = mean 2.84 – 0.85 = 1.99 and 2.84 + 0.85 = 3.69. The 99th CI = (1.99, 3.69).

$$99\text{th CI} = \text{mean} \pm 2.58\ SE_M = 2.84 \pm 2.58 \times 0.33 = 2.84 \pm 0.85 = (1.99, 3.69)$$

6. The term *double-blind* means that the subjects and the researchers were unaware of who was administered the treatments and who was given the placebo. In this case, the treatments consisted of 125 mg or 250 mg of bosentan twice a day (bid). The subjects were randomly assigned to either the 125 mg or 250 mg bosentan treatments groups or the placebo control group. Thus, the groups were randomly determined and the members of the placebo group were given an inactive form of the drug, which is why the researchers refer to this as the placebo-control group.
7. Null hypothesis: There is no difference between the combined bosentan arms and placebo group in the distributions of change from baseline in echocardiographic and doppler parameters. The term combined bosentan arms refers to both groups that were given the drug, where 56 subjects were given either 125 mg or 250mg of bosentan twice a day (bid).
8. For some of the variables, a negative change may be a desired result. For example, in the treatment groups there was a reduction in maximal tricuspid regurgitant velocity, which resulted in a negative number. Reducing this velocity is a desired effect of the medication, because a high velocity reflects a high blood flow through the heart, which leads to lesions and muscle atrophy. When diagnosing pulmonary artery hypertension, the tricuspid regurgitant velocity is one of the measurements recorded.
9. $SE_M = 0.10$ for IVC minimum diameter (cm) for the 250 mg bosentan group. 99th CI = 1.38 – 0.26 = 1.12 and 1.38 + 0.26 = 1.64. The 99th CI = (1.12, 1.64).

$$99\text{th CI} = \text{mean} \pm 2.58\ SE_M = 1.38 \pm 2.58(0.10) = 1.38 \pm 0.26 = (1.12, 1.64)$$

■ EXERCISE 34 Questions to be Graded

1. What were the mean and standard deviation for RV ejection time (ms) for the 125 mg of bosentan in the baseline Doppler group?

2. What were the mean and standard deviation for the Doppler MV peak E velocity (cm/s) in the bosentan groups combined?

3. Calculate the SE_M for Doppler RV index in the placebo group. Round your answer to two decimal places.

4. Calculate the SE_M for cardiac index in the bosentan groups combined. Round your answer to two decimal places.

5. Calculate the SE_M for Doppler MV E/A ratio in the placebo group. Round your answer to two decimal places.

6. Calculate the 99th CI for the doppler RV index in the placebo group. Round your answer to two decimal places.

7. Calculate the 99th CI for the doppler MV E/A ratio in the placebo group. Round your answer to two decimal places.

8. The researchers used two different dosages of the treatment drug, 125 mg and 250 mg of bosentan. What was the reason for this?

9. The article stated, "there was a trend towards a reduction of the maximal tricuspid regurgitant velocity in patients treated with bosentan, although the difference from the placebo group did not reach statistical significance" (Galiè et al., 2003, p. 1383). What do these findings mean, and are they useful in clinical practice? Provide a rationale for your answer.

10. Compare the means and standard deviations for heart rate (beats/min) in the placebo and the bosentan groups combined. What did you find? What effect did the treatment bosentan have on heart rate, and might this be clinically important? Provide a rationale for your answer.

STANDARD ERROR OF A PERCENTAGE AND 95TH CONFIDENCE INTERVAL

STATISTICAL TECHNIQUE IN REVIEW

When researchers use only a small sample of a population, or conduct research on a phenomenon over a short period of time, there is a sampling error because not all of the population is sampled. When a smaller percentage of the population is included in a study, the error will be larger (Burns & Grove, 2005). When analyzing the data, researchers can calculate the standard error of a percentage and the 95% confidence interval. This means that the true percentage for that population is somewhere in between the two numbers, and the chances are 95 out of 100 that the true percentage of the population lies within the confidence interval. To review percentages, see Exercises 4 and 5. The formula used for calculating the standard error of a percentage is:

$$S = \sqrt{\frac{pq}{n}}$$

Note: S = standard error of %
p = % found in the sample
$q = 100 - p$
n or N = sample size.
Example: $p = 35\%$ and $N = 100$.
Calculation: $S = \sqrt{35} \ (100 - 35) \div \sqrt{100} = 4.77$

RESEARCH ARTICLE

Source: Thomson, C. S., Brewster, D. H., Dewar, J. A., & Twelves, C. J. (2004). Improvements in survival for women with breast cancer in Scotland between 1987 and 1993: Impact of earlier diagnosis and changes in treatment. *European Journal of Cancer, 40*(5), 743–53.

Introduction

A study was conducted to compare the 8-year survival rates and causes in women diagnosed with breast cancer in 1987 and 1993. This study was conducted in Scotland. The subjects were women with early breast cancer who were "without metastases at diagnosis and who underwent surgery as part of their primary treatment" (Thompson et al., 2004, p. 743). The sample consisted of 1,617 women from 1987, and 2,077 who were diagnosed in 1993. The study results indicated that survival increased by 11% from 1987 to 1993, and that this increase was a result of screening and earlier diagnosis as well as improvements in treatments and heath care delivery in Scotland (Thomson et al., 2004).

Relevant Study Results

Earlier studies have shown that regional locality and specialization of the surgeon have an impact on survival. This represented a difference in treatment related to the socioeconomic status of the patient, which leads to decreased survival for those who were of a lower socioeconomic level or those who resided in areas with fewer resources. With this in mind, the government initiated a screening program, organized surgeons into surgical specialization, and reorganized the health care system to offer more adequate services. The years 1987 and 1993 were picked for this study because they reflect the changes that had been made in the health care delivery system.

The findings of the researchers were that there was a significant difference between the two groups in clinical/pathological prognostic factors. When diagnosed via screening, the tumors had better prognostic features, and the tumors detected in 1993 were more likely to be clinical stage I. When comparing adjuvant therapy for the two groups, 53.3% were given radiotherapy in 1993 compared with 41.3% in 1987. With chemotherapy, 18.6% were treated in 1993 and 7.7% in 1987. Endocrine therapy results were similar, with 92.4% in 1993 compared with 65.5% in 1987. Differences also related to surgeon caseload, number of patients seen by an oncologist, and those who were diagnosed via screening. Table 3 represents the survival estimates at 8 years for the clinical/pathological factors for the two cohorts, and Table 4 represents the univariate survival estimates at 8 years for the treatment and health care delivery/deprivation factors for the two cohorts. Differences between the two groups were also provided (Thomson et al., 2003).

TABLE 3 ■ Univariate Survival Estimates at 8 Years for the Clinical/Pathological Factors for the Two Cohorts

Clinical/pathological factors	8-YEAR FIGURE FOR 1987		8-YEAR FIGURE FOR 1993		DIFFERENCE (1993-1987)	
	Survival (%)	95% CI (%)	Survival (%)	95% CI (%)	Survival (%)	95% CI (%)
Age group (years)						
< 50	63.4	59.0–67.7	71.0	67.2–74.8	7.7	1.9–13.4
50–64	61.6	57.7–65.5	75.8	73.0–78.6	14.3	9.5–19.0
65–79	51.3	46.8–55.8	58.9	54.6–63.2	7.6	1.4–13.9
≥ 80	25.3	15.5–35.2	38.3	29.6–47.0	13.0	−0.1–26.1
Clinical stage[a]						
I	73.1	68.1–78.0	80.1	77.2–83.1	7.1	1.3–12.8
II	57.5	54.1–60.9	64.9	61.8–6,7.9	7.4	2.8–11.9
III	37.8	30.8–44.8	38.2	31.2–45.1	0.3	−9.6–10.2
Not known	53.2	47.7–58.8	70.0	64.2–75.8	16.8	8.7–24.8
ER status						
Positive	65.5	61.7–69.3	74.6	71.6–77.7	9.1	4.2–14.0
Negative	48.3	43.4–53.3	56.6	51.4–61.8	8.2	1.1–15.4
Not known	55.1	51.2–59.0	67.6	64.6–70.5	12.5	7.6–17.4
Pathological node status						
Positive	44.4	40.4–48.4	52.3	48.6–56.0	8.0	2.5–13.4
INS[b]	70.3	65.0–75.7	74.4	69.1–79.7	4.1	−3.4–11.6
Negative[c]	75.6	70.8–80.4	80.7	78.0–83.3	5.1	−0.4–10.6
Not known	53.7	49.1–58.4	64.3	58.7–70.0	10.6	3.3–17.9
Pathological tumor size						
≤ 2cm	67.1	63.5–70.8	77.7	75.3–80.1	10.6	6.2–14.9
> 2cm	48.6	44.8–52.4	55.0	51.3–58.7	6.3	1.0–11.6
Not known	56.0	50.5–61.5	61.7	55.5–68.0	5.7	−2.6–14.1

95% CI, 95% Confidence Interval.

[a] Clinical stage was determined prior to surgery at the time of presentation of the initial examination. This means that it will be related, but will not necessarily be identical, to the pathological staging information.

[b] INS = inadequate negative sample = 1, 2, 3, unknown number taken, all negative.

[c] Negative = four or more nodes taken, all negative.

Thomson, C. S., Brewster, D. H., Dewar, J. A., & Twelves, C. J. (2004). Improvements in survival for women with breast cancer in Scotland between 1987 and 1993: Impact of earlier diagnosis and changes in treatment. *European Journal of Cancer, 40*(5), p. 748.

TABLE 4 ■ Univariate Survival Estimates at 8 Years for the Treatment and Health Care Delivery/ Deprivation Factors for the Two Cohorts

	8-YEAR FIGURE FOR 1987		8-YEAR FIGURE FOR 1993		DIFFERENCE (1993–1987)	
	Survival (%)	95% CI (%)	Survival (%)	95% CI (%)	Survival (%)	95% CI (%)
Treatment factors						
Type of surgery						
Mastectomy	54.5	51.3–57.7	62.8	59.7–65.8	8.3	3.9–12.7
Breast conservation	61.5	57.8–65.2	73.2	70.6–75.8	11.6	7.1–16.2
Adjuvant radiotherapy						
Given	58.2	54.5–61.9	69.7	67.1–72.3	11.5	6.9–16.0
Not given	56.8	53.6–60.0	66.5	63.4–69.6	9.7	5.3–14.2
Adjuvant chemotherapy						
Given	48.4	39.6–57.2	62.0	57.2–66.9	13.6	3.6–23.7
Not given	58.1	55.6–60.6	69.8	67.6–72.0	11.6	8.3–15.0
Adjuvant endocrine therapy						
Given	56.5	53.5–59.4	68.3	66.2–70.4	11.8	8.2–15.4
Not given	59.1	55.1–63.2	68.8	61.5–76.0	9.6	1.3–18.0
Adjuvant systemic therapy (chemotherapy or endocrine therapy)						
Given	56.0	53.1–58.9	67.9	65.8–69.9	11.9	8.3–15.4
Not given	60.8	56.4–65.2	79.3	70.5–88.1	18.5	8.6–28.3
Health care delivery/ demographic/actors						
Health Board of Residence						
Ayrshire and Arran	48.2	39.7–56.6	67.9	60.8–74.9	19.7	8.7–30.7
Borders	58.1	40.7–75.4	80.0	69.4–90.6	21.9	1.6–42.3
Argyll and Clyde	48.2	39.8–56.5	75.9	69.9–81.9	27.7	17.4–38.0
Fife	61.2	52.5–69.8	72.2	64.0–80.4	11.0	−0.9–22.9
GGHB	58.7	53.0–64.5	64.7	59.5–69.9	6.0	−1.8–13.8
Highland	56.5	44.8–68.2	61.5	51.7–71.2	4.9	−10.3–20.2
Islands	60.0	42.5–77.5	67.4	53.4–81.5	7.4	−15.0–29.9
Lanarkshire	52.6	44.7–60.6	66.7	60.2–73.1	14.0	3.8–24.3
Grampian	59.3	52.1–66.6	67.2	60.6–73.8	7.9	−1.9–17.6
Lothian	69.2	63.0–75.4	68.9	63.6–74.2	−0.3	−8.4–7.9
Tayside	57.0	48.7–65.4	64.0	57.3–70.7	6.9	−3.8–17.6
Forth Valley	49.3	37.9–60.8	68.9	60.1–77.7	19.6	5.1–34.0
Dumfries and Galloway	60.0	48.1–71.9	75.3	65.9–84.7	15.3	0.1–30.5
Surgical case load[a]						
1–9 cases	52.4	46.5–58.3	53.8	46.6–60.9	1.4	−7.9–10.7
10–29	54.1	50.4–57.9	64.8	60.2–69.3	10.7	4.8–16.5
Team/ ≥ 30	63.3	59.6–67.0	71.3	68.9–73.6	7.9	3.6–12.3
Seen by oncologist[b]						
Yes	57.5	54.2–60.8	69.5	67.1–71.9	12.0	7.9–16.0
No	57.4	53.8–61.0	66.0	62.3–69.7	8.5	3.4–13.7
Deprivation category[c] 1991 Census						
Least	60.8	55.8–65.8	73.4	69.3–77.5	12.6	6.2–19.1
Intermediate	58.0	54.9–61.1	67.9	65.4–70.5	9.9	5.9–14.0
Most	50.9	45.0–56.7	63.1	58.0–68.2	12.2	4.4–19.9
Screen-detected?						
Yes	82.1	70.0–94.1	84.9	81.8–88.0	2.8	−9.6–15.3
No	56.8	54.3–59.2	62.8	60.4–65.2	6.1	2.6–9.5

[a]Note that the 12 and 13 cases for the 1987 and 1993 cohorts, respectively, where the surgeon was unknown were not included in the analyses.
[b] Note that the 29 and 22 cases for the 1987 and 1993 cohorts, respectively, where the date of referral to the oncologist was unknown were not included in the analyses, as it was not possible to determine if consultation was part of the primary treatment.
[c] Note that a deprivation score could not be assigned for 2 cases in the 1987 cohort.
ER equals Estrogen Receptor
Thomson, C. S., Brewster, D. H., Dewar, J. A., & Twelves, C. J. (2004). Improvements in survival for women with breast cancer in Scotland between 1987 and 1993: Impact of earlier diagnosis and changes in treatment. *European Journal of Cancer, 40*(5), p. 749.

■ STUDY QUESTIONS

1. In the 1987 group, which age range had the highest survival rate (percentage)?

2. In the 1993 group, what was the percentage of survival for women who had clinical stage III breast cancer at diagnosis?

3. What was the difference between the two groups (1987 and 1993) in survival percentage when the tumor was Estrogen Receptor (ER) positive?

4. Which Health Board of Residence had the lowest survival rate in 1987?

5. What surgical caseload provided the best outcome for the 1993 group? Provide a rationale for your answer.

6. The samples included 1,617 women in 1987 and 2,077 women in 1993. Why were more women diagnosed with breast cancer in 1993 than in 1987?

7. Examine the age groups. The lowest survival rate and the greatest difference in the confidence intervals (CI) are found in the over-80 age group. Provide a rationale for these results.

8. Deprivation category, or socioeconomic status, did not appear to have a major impact on the survival of women in the 1993 group. Provide a rationale for this result.

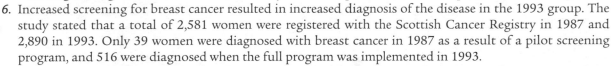

ANSWERS TO STUDY QUESTIONS

1. The < 50 age group had the highest survival rate at 63.4 % for the 1987 group (see Table 3).
2. 38.2% of the women with clinical stage III breast cancer at diagnosis survived for the 1993 group (see Table 3).
3. There was a 9.1% difference in survival from 1987 (65.5% survival) to 1993 (74.6% survival) (see Table 3).
4. Two Health Boards of Residences had the lowest survival rate for 1987 at 48.2%: Ayrshire and Arran, and Argyll and Clyde.
5. The surgical caseload of team ≥ 30 had the highest survival rate at 71.3%. Surgeons have greater proficiency with increased surgical cases. In addition, the team approach usually provides a stronger treatment plan based on the knowledge and expertise of the surgeons involved. The cancer treatment advancements listed in the article assisted the surgeon teams in improving care for patients. Those advancements were increased screening leading to earlier treatment, more adjuvant therapies, and increased specialization of surgeons.
6. Increased screening for breast cancer resulted in increased diagnosis of the disease in the 1993 group. The study stated that a total of 2,581 women were registered with the Scottish Cancer Registry in 1987 and 2,890 in 1993. Only 39 women were diagnosed with breast cancer in 1987 as a result of a pilot screening program, and 516 were diagnosed when the full program was implemented in 1993.
7. The survival percentage for the over-80 age group in 1987 was 25.3% with a 95% CI of 15.5–35.2, and the survival percentage for 1993 was 38.3% with a 95% CI of 29.6–47.0. These results indicate that women over 80 have the lowest survival rate. This result is expected, since older women have more fragile health conditions, are less likely to survive surgery, have more comorbid conditions, and might have more side effects with adjuvant therapies. The size of the CI indicates that a large difference in survival rates occurred in the over-80 age group, which could be due to the varied levels of health of this age group and their varied responses to therapies.
8. Table 4 shows a 73.4% survival in the least deprivation category and 63.1% in the most deprivation category for the 1993 group, a difference of 10.3%. The discrepancy in survival is somewhat limited since Scotland, like the rest of the United Kingdom, has socialized medicine. Socialized medicine provides access to care regardless of socioeconomic status; however, some rural areas in Scotland have limited access to care and often more disadvantaged individuals. The 10.3% survival difference between the patients in the least and most deprivation categories does indicate the two groups of patients were receiving different treatments. However, a major program was implemented in Scotland to improve the assessment, diagnosis, and treatment of women with breast cancer, so you would expect improved survival for women with breast cancer for all socioeconomic categories for 1993.

■ EXERCISE 35   Questions to be Graded

1. Identify the confidence interval (CI) for the women diagnosed with breast cancer in the 1993 group who were negative in all nodes.

2. What was the survival rate (percentage) for women diagnosed with breast cancer in the 1987 group who had unknown pathological tumor size?

3. What tumor size was related to the best survival percentage?

4. What was the difference in survival rate from the 1987 group to the 1993 group for the Health Board of Residence of Argyll and Clyde? How did this figure compare with the other Health Boards of Residence?

5. In comparing the 1987 and 1993 groups, which group was more likely to receive adjuvant therapies? Give your answers as percentages.

6. This study was conducted in Scotland. Can the findings be generalized to the United States?

The formula that is found in the review of statistical information for this exercise can be used to calculate the standard error of a percentage. This figure would then be added to and subtracted from the mean percent to arrive at the 95% CI. The researchers did not provide the sample size for each category in Tables 3 and 4, so for Questions 7, 8, and 9, use the sample size of 250 to do your calculations.

7. What was the standard error of a percentage for the < 50 age group for the 1987 group? Round your answer to two decimal places.

8. What was the standard error of a percentage for the Estrogen Receptor (ER) status positive in the 1987 group?

9. Use your answer from Question 8 to calculate the 95% confidence interval (CI) for Estrogen Receptor (ER) positive status in the 1987 group.

10. Review the results in Tables 3 and 4 and make a statement about the survival rates from the 1987 group to the 1993 group. Provide a brief rationale for these results.

36

ANALYSIS OF VARIANCE (ANOVA) I

STATISTICAL TECHNIQUE IN REVIEW

An **analysis of variance (ANOVA)** statistical technique is conducted to examine differences between two or more groups. There are different types of ANOVA, with the most basic being the **one-way ANOVA**, which is used to analyze data in studies with one independent and one dependent variable. More details on the types of ANOVA can be found in your research textbook and statistical texts (Burns & Grove, 2005; Munro, 2001). The outcome of ANOVA is a numerical value for the F statistic. The calculated F-ratio from ANOVA indicates the extent to which group means differ, taking into account the variability within the groups. Assuming the null hypothesis of no difference among groups is true; the probability of obtaining an F-ratio as large or larger than that obtained in the given sample is indicated by the calculated p value. For example, if $p = 0.0002$, this indicates that the probability of obtaining a result like this in future studies is rare, and one may conclude that group differences exist and the null hypothesis is rejected. However, there is always a possibility that this decision is in error, and the probability of committing this Type I error is determined by the alpha (α) set for the study, which is usually 0.05 that is smaller in health care studies and occasionally 0.01.

ANOVA is similar to the t-test since the null hypothesis (no differences between groups) is rejected when the analysis yields a smaller p value, such as $p \leq 0.05$, than the alpha set for the study. Assumptions for the ANOVA statistical technique include:

1. normal distribution of the populations from which the samples were drawn or random samples;
2. groups should be mutually exclusive;
3. groups should have equal variance or homogeneity of variance;
4. independence of observations;
5. dependent variable is measured at least at the interval level (Burns & Grove, 2005; Munro, 2001).

Researchers who perform ANOVA on their data record their results in an ANOVA summary table or in the text of a research article. An example of how an ANOVA result is commonly expressed is:

$$F_{(1, 343)} = 15.46, p < 0.001$$

Where:
F is the statistic
1 is the group degrees of freedom (df) calculated by $K - 1$, where K = number of groups in the study. In this example, $K - 1 = 2 - 1 = 1$.
343 is the error degrees of freedom (df) that is calculated based upon the number of participants or $N - K$. In this example, 345 subjects – 2 groups = 343 error df.
15.46 is the F ratio or value
p indicates the significance of the F ratio in this study or $p < 0.001$.

There are different types of ANOVA, but the focus of these analysis techniques is on examining differences between two or more groups. The simplest is the one-way ANOVA, but many of the studies in the literature include more complex ANOVA techniques. A commonly used ANOVA technique is the **repeated-measures analysis of variance**, which is used to analyze data from studies where the same variable(s) is (are) repeatedly measured over time on a group or groups of subjects. The intent is to determine the change that occurs over time in the dependent variable(s) with exposure to the independent treatment variable(s).

RESEARCH ARTICLE

Source: Baird, C. L., & Sands, L. (2004). A pilot study of the effectiveness of guided imagery with progressive muscle relaxation to reduce chronic pain and mobility difficulties of osteoarthritis. *Pain Management Nursing, 5*(3), 97–104.

Introduction

"Osteoarthritis (OA) is a common, chronic condition that affects most older adults. Adults with OA must deal with pain that leads to limited mobility and may lead to disability and difficulty maintaining independence" (Baird & Sands, 2004, p. 97). Baird and Sands (2004) conducted a longitudinal, randomized clinical trial pilot study "to determine whether Guided Imagery (GI) with Progressive Muscle Relaxation (PMR) would reduce pain and mobility difficulties of women with OA" (Baird & Sands, 2004, p. 97). The sample included 28 women over 65: 18 women were randomly assigned to the intervention group, and 10 were randomly assigned to the control group. "The treatment consisted of listening twice a day to a 10-to-15 minute audiotaped script that guided the women in GI with PMR. Repeated measures ANOVA revealed a significant difference between the two groups in the amount of change in pain and mobility difficulties they experienced over 12 weeks. The treatment group reported a significant reduction in pain and mobility difficulties at week 12 compared to the control group. Members of the control group reported no differences in pain and nonsignificant increases in mobility difficulties. The results of this pilot study justify further investigation of the effectiveness of GI with PMR as a self-management intervention to reduce pain and mobility difficulties associated with OA" (Baird & Sands, 2004, p. 97).

Relevant Study Results

"Repeated-measures ANOVA revealed a significant difference between the two groups in how much change in pain they experienced for 12 weeks ($F_{[1, 26]} = 4.406$, $p = 0.046$). The 17 participants in the intervention group reported a significant reduction in pain ($p < 0.001$) at week 12 compared to the control group, whose members reported no change in their pain at week 12 (see Figure 1)" (Baird & Sands, 2004, p. 100).

FIGURE 1 ■ Change in pain over 12 weeks. Pain was significantly less in the guided imagery intervention group ($p = .046$).

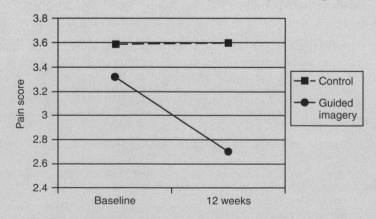

Baird, C. L., & Sands, L. (2004). A pilot study of the effectiveness of guided imagery with progressive muscle relaxation to reduce chronic pain and mobility difficulties of osteoarthritis. *Pain Management Nursing, 5*(3), p. 101. Copyright © 2004, with permission from the American Society for Pain Management Nursing.

"Repeated-measures ANOVA revealed a significant difference between the two groups in how much change in mobility the women experienced over the 12 weeks ($F_{(1, 22)} = 9.619$, $p = 0.005$). The participants in the intervention group reported a significant reduction in mobility difficulty at week 12 ($p < 0.001$). In contrast, those in the control group actually had increases in mobility difficulty at week 12, although these increases did not reach statistical significance (see Figure 2)" (Baird & Sands, 2004, p. 101).

FIGURE 2 ■ Change in mobility difficulties over 12 weeks. Mobility difficulties were significantly less in the guided imagery intervention group ($p = .005$).

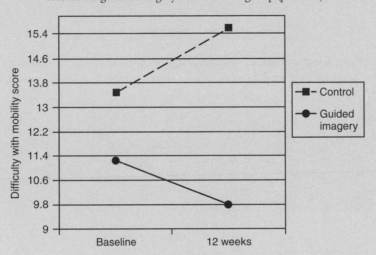

■ STUDY QUESTIONS

1. What type of analysis was conducted in this study? Was this analysis technique appropriate? Provide a rationale for your answer.

2. According to Figure 1, at which time was the average pain score for the guided imagery group most similar to the control group? Discuss the importance of this finding.

3. Discuss what each aspect of this result means: $F_{(1, 26)} = 4.406, p = 0.046$.

4. Is the change in the pain scores after 12 weeks of guided imagery statistically significant for the intervention group? If yes, at what probability?

5. State the null hypothesis for the effect of guided imagery on pain scores for the subjects in the treatment group at 12 weeks. Should this null hypothesis be accepted or rejected? Provide a rationale for your answer.

6. How many means are being compared for the pain scores at 12 weeks?

7. What did the researcher set the level of significance or alpha (α) at for this study? When will study results be considered significant?

8. The researchers do not report the standard deviations associated with the means. Would you be interested in knowing the standard deviations? Provide a rationale for your answer.

■ ANSWERS TO STUDY QUESTIONS

1. A repeated-measures ANOVA was conducted to examine differences between the intervention group, receiving the treatment of GI and the control group over 12 weeks. The groups were examined for differences for the dependent variables of pain and mobility over the 12-week time period. The repeated-measures ANOVA was appropriate since the focus was on examining group differences over time. In addition, the groups were independent due to random group assignment, and the dependent variables (pain and mobility) were measured at least at the interval level of measurement.

2. According to Figure 1, the average pain scores for the guided imagery intervention group and the control group were most similar at baseline. This is what the researchers would hope for, since they had a sample of 28 subjects who were randomly assigned to the treatment and control groups to promote similarity of the groups at the start of the study. Thus if a change occurred between the two groups during the study, it is assumed it is due to the treatment and not because the groups were different at the start of the study.

3. $F_{(1, 26)}$ = 4.406, p = 0.046, where F is the statistic for ANOVA and the group df = 1 and the error df = 26. The F ratio or value = 4.406, which is significant at p = 0.046

4. Yes, $F_{(1, 26)}$ = 4.406, p = 0.046 is statistically significant at p = 0.046. The level of significance for this study was set at α = 0.05, and since p is < this value, the study results are statistically significant.

5. The null hypothesis is: Women with OA receiving guided imagery have no greater improvement in their pain scores than those in the control group at 12 weeks. The study results indicated a significant improvement in the pain scores of women with OA who received the treatment of guided imagery ($F_{(1, 26)}$ = 4.406, p = 0.046). Thus, the null hypothesis was rejected.

6. Two means are being compared at 12 weeks. The mean of the control group and the mean of the guided imagery group for pain are being compared at 12 weeks.

7. The researchers set the level of significance or alpha (α) = 0.05, which means that any results with a p (probability) of ≤ 0.05 will be considered significant.

8. Answers may vary, but it would be helpful to include the standard deviations with the means since the standard deviations indicate the spread of the scores for the two groups. The standard deviations for the treatment and control groups also are needed to calculate the effect size or the effect of the treatment in a study. The effect size is needed to conduct a power analysis to predict the sample size needed for future studies. In addition, if the results from this study were to be combined with the results from other studies, the means and standard deviations for the treatment and control groups are needed to conduct a meta-analysis to combine study results to determine current knowledge in an area. In summary, it is helpful to report all means and standard deviations for study variables whether the results are significant or nonsignificant, because they are valuable to consider in conducting future research and meta-analyses.

■ EXERCISE 36   Questions to be Graded

1. The researchers found a significant difference between the two groups (control and treatment) for change in mobility of the women with osteoarthritis (OA) over 12 weeks with the results of $F_{(1, 22)} = 9.619$, $p = 0.005$. Discuss each aspect of these results.

2. State the null hypothesis for the Baird and Sands (2004) study that focuses on the effect of the GI with PMR treatment on patients' mobility level. Should the null hypothesis be rejected for the difference between the two groups in change in mobility scores over 12 weeks? Provide a rationale for your answer.

3. The researchers stated that the participants in the intervention group reported a reduction in mobility difficulty at week 12. Was this result statistically significant, and if so at what probability?

4. If the researchers had set the level of significance or $\alpha = 0.01$, would the results of $p = 0.001$ still be statistically significant? Provide a rationale for your answer.

5. If $F_{(3, 60)} = 4.13$, $p = 0.04$, and $\alpha = 0.01$, is the result statistically significant? Provide a rationale for your answer. Would the null hypothesis be accepted or rejected?

6. Can ANOVA be used to test proposed relationships or predicted correlations between variables in a single group? Provide a rationale for your answer.

7. If a study had a result of $F_{(2, 147)} = 4.56$, $p = 0.003$, how many groups were in the study, and what was the sample size?

8. The researchers state that the sample for their study was 28 women with a diagnosis of OA, and that 18 were randomly assigned to the intervention group and 10 were randomly assigned to the control group. Discuss the study strengths and/or weaknesses in this statement.

9. In your opinion, have the researchers established that guided imagery (GI) with progressive muscle relaxation (PMR) reduces pain and decreases mobility difficulties in women with OA?

10. The researchers stated that this was a 12-week longitudinal, randomized clinical trial pilot study with 28 women over 65 years of age with the diagnosis of OA. What are some of the possible problems or limitations that might occur with this type of study?

37

ANALYSIS OF VARIANCE (ANOVA) II

STATISTICAL TECHNIQUE IN REVIEW

There are different types of ANOVA, but the focus of this statistical technique is on examining differences between two or more groups. The one-way ANOVA is conducted when differences are examined for a study that has one independent variable and one dependent variable. The **two-way ANOVA** is conducted when differences are examined in a study that has two independent variables and one dependent variable. The **multivariate analysis of variance (MANOVA)** is conducted when a study has more than one independent and dependent variables. **Repeated measures analysis of variance** is used to analyze data from studies where the same variable(s) are repeatedly measured over time in a group or groups of subjects. The intent is to determine the change that occurs over time in the dependent variable(s) with the exposure to the independent variable(s). More details on the types of ANOVA can be found in your research and statistical texts (Burns & Grove, 2005; Munro, 2001).

RESEARCH ARTICLE

Source: Stevens, S. L., Colwell, B., Smith, D. W., Robinson, J., & McMillan, C. (2005). An exploration of self-reported negative affect by adolescents as a reason for smoking: Implications for tobacco prevention and intervention programs. *Preventive Medicine, 41*(2), 589–96.

Introduction

Stevens et al. (2005) conducted a study to investigate the differences between two groups of youth, those who had a negative affect reported and those who did not, on their smoking behaviors, attitudes, and self-efficacy. This study was conducted to "shed light on differences in adolescent smoking maintenance and cessation" based on their affect. "721 [*N* = 721] smoking youth participated in a cognitive-behavioral smoking cessation program. Reasons for smoking were categorized, and youth were placed into one of two groups based on presence or absence of negative affect. One-way ANOVA determined if differences existed on Fagerstrom Nicotine Tolerance Dependence (FNTD) scores" (Stevens et al., 2005, p. 589).

Relevant Study Results

"For future intentions, one-way repeated measures ANOVA revealed a significant main effect pre- to post-program on number of days intended to smoke in the next 30 ($F_{(1, 449)} = 7.98, p = 0.005$) and age intended quit ($F_{(1, 320)} = 7.51, p = 0.006$). Those reporting negative affect intended to smoke more days in the next 30 days and reported a higher intended age of quit than those not reporting negative affect as a reason for use (Table 2)" (Stevens et al., 2005, p. 593).

"One-way analysis of variance revealed no significant differences on pre-program FTND scores between the two groups ($F_{(1, 715)} = 3.128$, $p = 0.077$ [or 0.08 as in Table 2]. The group not reporting negative affect had a slightly higher dependent score (mean = 3.53; SD = 2.65) than the group self-reporting negative affect (mean = 3.18; SD = 2.46) (Table 2). According to the FTND scale, however, these scores indicate that neither group is very dependent on nicotine" (Stevens et al., 2005, p. 593).

"There were significant pre- to post-program main effects for the following attitude items: 'Smoking makes me look older' ($F_{(1, 517)} = 17.02$, $p < 0.001$); 'Smoking helps me make and keep friends' ($F_{(1, 517)} = 11.05$, $p = 0.001$); and 'Smoking helps me be accepted' ($F_{(1, 518)} = 9.86$, $p = 0.002$), with both groups agreeing more with these statements from pre- to post-programs (Table 2) … Significant main effects ($F_{(1, 500)} = 3.86$, $p = .05$) and significant group by time interaction ($F_{(1, 500)} = 6.08$, $p = 0.014$) for overall self-efficacy were demonstrated, with the negative affect group decreasing and the non-negative affect group increasing in self-efficacy from pre- to post-program (Table 2). Additionally, significant main effects for the following self-efficacy items were noted pre- to post-program: 'I believe I can quit if I try' ($F_{(1, 499)} = 9.13$, $p = 0.003$); and 'I have the skills necessary to quit' ($F_{(1, 498)} = 12.10$, $p = 0.001$), with both groups increasing in agreement with these items. Significant group by time interaction was found from pre- to post-program on the items: 'Quitting would be easy' ($F_{(1, 499)} = 6.10$, $p = 0.014$), with the group reporting negative affect as a reason for smoking decreasing in agreement with this item, and the group not reporting negative affect agreeing more; and on item: 'I can quit using anytime I want' ($F_{(1, 500)} = 7.70$, $p = 0.006$), with the group reporting negative affect as a reason for smoking agreeing less with this item and the group not reporting negative affect agreeing more. There was no significance for the following self-efficacy item: 'I can resist peer pressure to use' (Table 2)" (Stevens et al., 2005, pp. 593–4).

TABLE 2 ■ Comparisons Among Youth for Tobacco use Behaviors, Attitudes, and Self-efficacy					
	GROUP 1, NEGATIVE AFFECT REPORTED		GROUP 2, NEGATIVE AFFECT NOT REPORTED		
Variable	Pre-mean *(SD)*	Post-mean *(SD)*	Pre-mean *(SD)*	Post-mean *(SD)*	*P*
TOBACCO USE BEHAVIORS					
No. smoked daily	11.01 (9.04)	11.06 (9.08)	11.83 (9.75)	11.39 (9.58)	0.476
No. days smoked in past 30	22.15 (11.59)	22.43 (11.57)	22.36 (12.01)	22.39 (12.88)	0.726
No. days intend to smoke in next 30	20.95 (12.30)	20.37 (13.09)	20.28 (13.22)	17.96 (13.40)	0.005*
Age of intended quit	26.38 (19.84)	24.31 (14.67)	23.24 (13.89)	20.54 (9.11)	0.006*
ATTITUDES					
Over all attitude score	2.74 (0.517)	2.71 (0.580)	2.74 (0.517)	2.69 (0.577)	0.10
Smoking is very enjoyable	2.15 (0.845)	2.27 (0.953)	2.16 (0.910)	2.18 (0.981)	0.08
Smoking makes me look older	3.14 (0.755)	2.97 (0.846)	3.15 (0.684)	2.99 (0.867)	0.001*
Helps me make and keep friends	3.42 (0.618)	3.28 (0.772)	3.44 (0.607)	3.33 (0.773)	0.001*
Smoking helps me be accepted	3.36 (0.682)	3.22 (0.799)	3.40 (0.662)	3.29 (0.845)	0.002*
Smoking is relaxing	1.92 (0.821)	1.98 (0.942)	1.83 (0.858)	1.81 (0.892)	0.62
Like to think of myself as a smoker	2.51 (0.897)	2.56 (0.978)	2.55 (0.882)	2.56 (0.978)	0.44
SELF-EFFICACY					
Overall efficacy score	2.44 (0.855)	2.46 (0.866)	2.58 (0.810)	2.45 (0.810)	0.05*
I believe I can quit smoking if I try	2.11 (1.02)	2.05 (1.06)	2.25 (1.02)	2.03 (0.999)	0.003*
Quiting smoking would be easy	3.27 (1.27)	3.38 (1.25)	3.54 (1.25)	3.40 (1.32)	0.73
I have the skills necessary to quit	2.20 (0.982)	2.04 (0.940)	2.30 (0.942)	2.16 (0.953)	0.001*
I can quit using anytime I want	2.65 (1.16)	2.77 (1.23)	2.88 (1.26)	2.72 (1.23)	0.68
I can resist peer pressure to use	2.01 (1.08)	2.06 (1.04)	1.94 (1.03)	1.93 (1.01)	0.67
FTND SCORE	3.18 (2.46)		3.53 (2.66)		0.08

*Statistical significance at least at $p \leq 0.05$ level

Stevens, S. L., Colwell, B., Smith, D. W., Robinson, J., & McMillan, C. (2005). An exploration of self-reported negative affect by adolescents as a reason for smoking: Implications for tobacco prevention and intervention programs. Reprinted from *Preventive Medicine*, *41*(2), p. 593, with permission of Elsevier.

■ STUDY QUESTIONS

1. On average, did the participants in Group 1 or Group 2 report more cigarettes smoked daily? Provide a rationale for your answer.

2. According to Table 2, which of the following statements about the difference between Group 1 and Group 2 on the attitude "Smoking is very enjoyable" is true? Provide a rationale for your answer.
   a. Sampling error probably did not create the difference between the means.
   b. Sampling error probably did create the difference between the means.

3. What type of ANOVA was conducted to examine the main effect pre- to post-program on number of days intended to smoke in the next 30 ($F_{(1, 449)} = 7.98, p = 0.005$)? What is the focus of this type of ANOVA?

4. Should the null hypothesis be rejected for "I believe I can quit smoking if I try"? Provide a rationale for your answer.

5. What were the results (means, SDs, F value, and p value) for the age intended to quit smoking? Provide your interpretation of what these results mean.

6. In Table 2, how many of the comparisons between Groups 1 and 2 were not statistically significant? Provide a rationale for your answer.

7. Was the difference between Group 1 and Group 2 on overall efficacy scores statistically significant? At what level of alpha could one reject the null hypothesis for this result?

8. Which of the seven attitudes was (were) statistically significant at the strongest level? Provide a rationale for your answer.

9. The result for "Smoking makes me look older" was $F_{(1, 517)}$ = 17.02, $p < 0.001$. Using this result, identify how many groups were examined in this analysis and the number of participants. Provide a rationale for your answer. If needed, refer to Exercise 36.

■ ANSWERS TO STUDY QUESTIONS

1. The participants in Group 2 reported more cigarettes smoked, with a mean of 11.83 pre-program and 11.39 cigarettes post-program, than the participants in Group 1, who reported a mean of 11.01 cigarettes smoked pre-program and 11.06 cigarettes post-program.
2. b.   Sampling error probably did create the difference between the means. The result for "Smoking is very enjoyable" is not statistically significant with $p = 0.08$ since p is greater than $\alpha = 0.05$. When results are not statistically significant, differences between the groups are assumed to be random error and not related to the effects of the treatment.
3. A one-way repeated measures ANOVA was conducted to determine this study result as indicated in the narrative of the article. A one-way ANOVA is used to examine differences in a study that has one independent and one dependent variable. A repeated measures ANOVA is conducted to examine differences in means obtained from repeatedly measuring the same variable over time for two groups of subjects. Thus, the one-way repeated measures ANOVA was used to examine differences over time between the two groups, negative affect reported and negative affect not reported, for the dependent variable number of days intended to smoke in the next 30 pre- and post-program.
4. Yes. The null hypothesis should be rejected for "I believe I can quite smoking if I try" since the results were $F_{(1, 499)} = 9.13, p = 0.003$. The $p = 0.003$ indicates the results are statistically significant for the two groups since it is greater than $\alpha = 0.05$. The null hypothesis is rejected with significant results.
5. The one-way repeated measures ANOVA result for age intended to quit smoking was $F_{(1, 320)} = 7.51$, $p = 0.006$, and the means and SDs for pre- and post program for the negative affect reported group were 26.38 (19.84) and 24.31 (14.67), respectively, and pre- and post-program for the negative affect not reported group were 23.24 (13.89) and 20.54 (9.11), respectively. In this study, there was a statistically significant difference between the two groups over time for the age the subjects intended to quit smoking. The mean ages post-program indicate that the negative affect not reported group, or the group with a more positive affect, intended to quit smoking earlier or at age 20.54, versus the group with the negative affect reported,

who intended to stop smoking at age 24.31. In this study, there is a link between the age one will quit smoking and the subjects' affect.

6. According to Table 2, 10 comparisons between Groups 1 and 2 were not statistically significant. The p values for these variables are all > 0.05, which means the results are not statistically significant. Also, the significant p values have an * next to them, indicating statistical significance between the two groups for these variables, and those without an * indicate that the two groups are not significantly different for these variables.

7. Yes. The overall efficacy scores were statistically significant at $p = 0.05*$, as indicated in Table 2. This p value is statistically significant since it is equal to alpha at 0.05, and the null hypothesis would be rejected for overall efficacy scores. If the p value is equal to or less than ($\leq$) alpha, the null hypothesis is rejected.

8. The attitudes "Smoking makes me look older" and "Helps me make and keep friends" were both statistically significant at $p = 0.001$, which was the most significant p value since it was the smallest p value for the attitudes examined in the study.

9. The values (1, 517) are the degrees of freedom (df), with the 1 being group df and the 517 being the error df that can be used to determine the number of groups and sample size for that analysis. Refer to Exercise 36 for determination of the df in ANOVA. There were 2 groups (K) (negative affect reported and the negative affect not reported) studied ($K - 1 = 1$ group df). The sample size for this analysis was $N = 519$ participants, where $N - K = 517$, therefore $519 - 2 = 517$.

■ **EXERCISE 37** Questions to be Graded

1. Post-program on average, did the participants in Group 1 or Group 2 report more number of days they intended to smoke in the next 30? Provide a rationale for your answer.

2. Should the null hypothesis be rejected for the self-efficacy statement "Quitting smoking would be easy"? Provide a rationale for your answer.

3. In Table 2, how many of the comparisons between Group 1 and Group 2 produced statistically significant results? Provide a rationale for your answer.

4. Was the difference between Groups 1 and 2 on FTND scores statistically significant? If so, at what level of significance? What do these results mean according to the Relevent Study Results?

5. What type of analysis was conducted to examine the means for the pre-program FTND scores for differences? Was this analysis appropriate? Provide a rationale for your answer.

6. According to Table 2, which of the following statements about the difference between Groups 1 and 2 on the attitude "Helps me make and keep friends" is accurate? Provide a rationale for your answer.
   a. Sampling error probably did not create the difference between the means.
   b. Sampling error probably did create the difference between the means.

7. In this study, the result for the attitude "Smoking helps me be accepted" was $F_{(1, 518)} = 9.86, p < 0.002$. From this ANOVA result, determine how many groups were studied and how many participants were included in this analysis. Provide a rationale for your answer.

8. The headings for the columns in Table 2 are "Pre-mean and Post-mean." Why were means calculated instead of medians or modes? Provide a rationale for your answer.

9. Do you think the study results support the observations that adolescents are more likely to increase smoking and continue smoking longer because of a negative attitude? Provide a rationale for your answer.

10. Can the findings from this study be generalized to the target population of adolescent smokers? Provide a rationale for your answer.

38

POST HOC ANALYSES
FOLLOWING ANOVA

STATISTICAL TECHNIQUE IN REVIEW

When a significant *F* value is obtained from the conduct of ANOVA, additional analyses are needed to determine the specific location of the differences in a study with more than two groups. **Post hoc analyses** were developed to determine where the differences lie since some of the groups might be different and others might be similar. For example, a study might include three groups, an experimental group (receiving a treatment), placebo group (receiving a pseudo or false treatment such as a sugar pill in a drug study), and a comparison group (receiving standard care). The ANOVA resulted in a significant *F* ratio or value, but post hoc analyses are needed to determine the exact location of the differences. With post hoc analyses, researchers might find that the experimental group is significantly different than both the placebo and comparison groups but the placebo and comparison groups were not significantly different from each other. One could conduct three *t*-tests to determine differences among the three groups, but that would inflate the Type I error. A Type I error occurs when the results indicate that two groups are significantly different when in actuality the groups are not different. Thus, post hoc analyses were developed to detect the differences following ANOVA in studies with more than two groups to prevent an inflation of a Type I error. The frequently used post hoc analyses include Bonferroni correction, the Newman-Keuls test, the Tukey Honestly Significant Difference (HSD) test, the Scheffe test, and the Dunnett test (Burns & Grove, 2005).

With post hoc analyses, the alpha level is reduced in proportion to the number of additional tests required to locate the statistically significant differences. As the alpha level is decreased, reaching the level of significance becomes increasingly more difficult. With the Bonferroni correction, alpha is divided by the number of comparisons to be made. In the preceding example, three comparisons were made with the three groups (experimental and placebo, experimental and comparison, and placebo and comparison), thus $\alpha = 0.05 \div 3 = 0.0167$. For significance to occur, the *p* values must be ≤ 0.0167 versus 0.05. The Newman-Keuls test compares all possible pairs of means and is the most liberal of the post hoc tests discussed here. "Liberal" indicates that the alpha is not as severely decreased. The Tukey HSD test computes one value with which all means within the data set are compared. It is considered more stringent than the Newman-Keuls test and requires approximately equal samples sizes in each group. The most conservative test is the Scheffe, but with the decrease in Type I error there is an increase in Type II error, which is saying something is not significant when it is. The Dunnett test requires a control group, and the experimental groups are compared with the control group without a decrease in alpha (Burns & Grove, 2005).

RESEARCH ARTICLE 1

Source: Adams, M. A., Pelletier, R. L., Zive, M. M., & Sallis, J. F. (2005). Salad bars and fruit and vegetable consumption in elementary schools: A plate waste study. *Journal of the American Dietetic Association, 105*(11), 1789–92.

Introduction

The American Dietetic Association has recommended that people eat at least five servings of fruits and vegetables every day, but American children on average eat only three and a half servings per day. Salad bars are recommended as a way to increase fruit and vegetable consumption, but inadequate research has been conducted to examine their effectiveness. Therefore, Adams et al. conducted a study "to determine whether students attending schools with self-service salad bars consume a greater amount of fruits and vegetables compared with students using proportioned servings" (Adams et al., 2005, p. 1789). On post hoc analysis, they also evaluated the relationship between the number of items offered and fruit and vegetable consumption.

Relevant Study Results

"Students who attended schools with salad bars present took 112 ± 70 g fruits and vegetables on average compared with 104 ± 86 g taken by students at non-salad bar schools. These differences were not statistically significant. . . . The mean amounts consumed were also not significantly different between serving type (47 ± 60 g vs. 43 ± 58 g, respectively). Significant difference was found in schools with fruit and vegetable variety ($F = 2.83$, $p \leq 0.05$). The number of items offered varied by school with the two salad bar schools offering four and seven items each, and the preportioned schools offering five items each." (Adams et al. 2005, p. 1791.) The Tukey post hoc analysis test was conducted to examine differences in fruit and vegetable consumption among the high and low variety schools. A difference was suggested "in consumption between students in the highest and lowest variety schools ($p = 0.06$). A trend in increasing consumption [of fruits and vegetables] was noticed as variety increased. Fruit and vegetable weights adjusted for sex and grade levels are presented in Table 2." (Adams et al., 2005, p. 1791.)

TABLE 2 ■ Adjusted Mean Weights of Fruits and Vegetables Taken and Consumed by First–Through Fifth-Grade Students in Four California Schools (*n*=288)

Serving type	No. of students	Items served *(n)*	Items taken *(g)*	Items consumed *(g)*	Items consumed *(%)*
	←		Mean ± SE[a]		→
DISTRICT 1					
Preportioned school 1	76	5	96 ± 10	49 ± 7	51
Preportioned school 2	65	5	96 ± 12	38 ± 8	40
DISTRICT 2					
Salad bar school 1	70	4	117 ± 10	36 ± 7	31
Salad bar school 2	77	7	107 ± 10	61 ± 7	57

[a]SE = Standard error
Adams, M. A., Pelletier, R. L., Zive, M. M., & Sallis, J. F. (2005). Salad bars and fruit and vegetable consumption in elementary schools: A plate waste study. *Journal of the American Dietetic Association, 105*(11), p. 1791. Copyright © 2005, with permission from The American Dietetic Association.

■ STUDY QUESTIONS

1. Adams et al. (2005) found no significant differences in the fruits and vegetables taken by students who were in schools with or without salad bars. Was a post hoc analysis conducted for this study result? Provide a rationale for your answer.

2. Did Adams et al. (2005) perform a post hoc analysis in their study? Provide a rationale for your answer.

3. What post hoc analysis was conducted in this study? Was this post hoc test more liberal or stringent than the Newman-Keuls test? Provide a rationale for your answer.

4. Could the Dunnett test have been conducted to determine differences in the schools? Provide a rationale for your answer.

5. Did the schools offering salad bars or the schools offering preportioned fruits and vegetables have more items taken by the students?

6. Which school consumed the most fruit and vegetable items, and what was the percentage of items consumed?

7. What school consumed the least items, and what was the percentage of items consumed?

8. Explain how the researchers were able to conclude from the results that "a trend in increasing fruit and vegetable consumption was noticed as variety increased" (Adams et al., 2005, p. 1791).

9. Did the students in schools with salad bars take more fruits and vegetables than those students in schools without salad bars? Do these study findings support putting salad bars in schools?

◼ ANSWERS TO STUDY QUESTIONS

1. No, a post hoc analysis was not performed for this result since it was not significant. Post hoc analysis is conducted for significant ANOVA results to determine the specific location of group differences.

2. Yes, Adams et al. (2005) did perform a post-hoc analysis in their study since they found a significant difference among schools with fruit and vegetable variety offered ($F = 2.83, p \leq 0.05$). The study included a number of schools with different variety in the fruits and vegetables offered. Thus, a post hoc analysis was conducted to determine the exact location of the differences among the schools without inflating the Type I error.

3. The Tukey HSD test was conducted, and it is considered more stringent than the Newman-Keuls test (Burns & Grove, 2005). The Tukey HSD test computes one value with which all the means in the data set are compared, whereas the Newman-Keuls compares all the possible pairs of means, which can increase the chance of a Type I error.

4. No, the Dunnett test could not have been conducted as a post hoc analysis in this study since there was no control group. The Dunnett test requires comparison of experimental groups with a control group.

5. The two schools in District 2, which had salad bars, had more fruit and vegetable items taken (means of 117 and 107) than the schools in District 1, which had preportioned fruits and vegetables (both with means of 96) (see Table 2 from Research Article 1).

6. In District 2, Salad bar school 2 was where students consumed the most amount of fruit and vegetable items, which was 61 items or 57%.

7. In District 2, Salad bar school 1 was where students consumed the least amount of fruit and vegetable items, which was 36 items or 31%.

8. The schools with salad bars that had the greatest variety of fruit and vegetable items offered also had the highest mean amounts of fruit and vegetables consumed, where the school with the lowest variety of items offered had the lowest consumption. Although $p = 0.06$ is not a statistically significant difference since it is greater than $\alpha = 0.05$, the researchers discussed the results as a trend since the results were close to being significant.

9. There was no statistically significant difference in the fruits and vegetables taken by students in schools with salad bars versus schools without salad bars. The findings do not support the use of salad bars in schools to increase the number of fruits or vegetables taken by the students. The results in the study supported that the variety of the items offered increased the consumption, but this was only a trend ($p = 0.06$). Additional research is needed to determine the impact of salad bars on student consumption of fruits and vegetables. This is an important area of research since nutrition makes a major contribution to health.

RESEARCH ARTICLE 2

 Source: Zampelas, A., Panagiotakos, D. B., Pitsavos, C., Das, U. N., Chrysohoou, C., Skoumas, Y., & Stefanadis, C. (2005). Fish consumption among healthy adults is associated with decreased levels of inflammatory markers related to cardiovascular disease: The ATTICA study. *Journal of the American College of Cardiology, 46*(1), 120–4.

Introduction

The consumption of fish has been associated with reduced risk of coronary heart disease, but the mechanisms have not been well investigated. Thus, Zampelas et al. investigated "the association between fish consumption and levels of various inflammatory markers among adults without any evidence of cardiovascular disease" (2005, p. 120). The study was a "cross-sectional survey that enrolled 1,541 men (age 18 to 87 years) and 1,528 women (age 18 to 89 years) from the Attica region, Greece. Of them, 5% of men and 3% of women were excluded due to a history of cardiovascular disease. Among others, C-reactive protein (CRP), interleukin (IL)-6, tumor necrosis factor (TNF)-alpha, serum amyloid A (SAA), and white blood cells (WBC) were measured, and dietary habits (including fish consumption) were evaluated using a validated food frequency questionnaire. A total of 88% of men and 91% of women reported fish consumption at least once a month. . . . Fish consumption was independently associated with lower inflammatory markers levels, among healthy adults. The strength and consistency of this finding has implications for public health and should be explored further" (Zampelas et al., 2005, p. 120).

Relevant Study Results

"All inflammatory markers showed an inverse dose-response relationship with fish consumption (Table 2). Based on the applied post hoc analysis, more prominent differences were observed when we compared high fish intake (i.e., > 300 g per week) with no consumption. Particularly, compared to non-fish consumers, those who consumed > 300 g of fish per week had on average 33% lower CRP, 33% lower IL-6, 21% lower TNF-alpha, 28% lower SAA levels, and 4% lower WBC counts (all $p < 0.05$)" (Zampelas et al., 2005, p. 121). The researchers also found significant differences when lower quantities (150 to 300 g/week) of fish were consumed.

An ANOVA was conducted among the 4 fish consumptions groups (no consumption, <150 g/week, 150–300 g/week, and > 300 g/week) to detect significant differences among these groups. Since the initial results were significant, the Bonferroni correction was conducted to detect exactly where the differences exist among the 4 study groups without inflating the Type I error (see Table 2 from Research Article 2).

TABLE 2 ■ Inflammatory Markers and Daily Fish Consumption

	FISH CONSUMPTION				
	No.	<150 g/week	150-300 g/week	>300 g/week	*p* Value
Number of participants (%)	319 (11%)	1,719 (56%)	745 (24%)	259 (9%)	–
C-reactive protein (mg/l)	2.7 ± 1.2	2.0 ± 1.1[†]	2.0 ± 2.1[†]	1.8 ± 1.1[†]	0.004
Interleukin-6 (ng/ml)	1.5 ± 0.5	1.3 ± 0.6[‡]	1.2 ± 1.1[†]	1.0 ± 0.3[†]	0.03
Tumor necrosis factor-alpha (mg/dl)	5.3 ± 3	5.1 ± 2	4.7 ± 3[†]	4.2 ± 2[†]	<0.001
Amyloid A (mg/dl)	6.4 ± 4	5.9 ± 4	5.1 ± 4[‡]	4.6 ± 3[†]	0.004
White blood cells (× 1.000 counts)	6.8 ± 3	6.7 ± 4	6.5 ± 4[‡]	6.5 ± 3[‡]	0.04

No gender differences were observed. *p = values derived from ANOVA that evaluated the associations between inflammatory markers (dependent) and fish intake (independent factor). [‡]$p < 0.05$ and [†]$p < 0.01$ (Bonferroni-corrected) for the differences between fish consumption groups vs. no consumption. Probability values derived from the analysis of variance (ANOVA).

Zampelas, A., Panagiotakos, D., Pitsavos, C., Das, U., Chrysohoou, C., Skoumas, Y., & Stefanadis, C. (2005). Fish consumption among healthy adults is associated with decreased levels of inflammatory markers related to cardiovascular disease. *Journal of the American College of Cardiology, 46*(1), p. 122. Copyright © 2005, with permission from The American College of Cardiology Foundation.

■ EXERCISE 38   Questions to be Graded:

1. When is a post hoc analysis performed in a study?

2. Did Zampelas et al. (2005) perform a post hoc analysis in their study? Provide a rationale for your answer.

3. What post hoc analysis was conducted in this study? Was this post hoc test more liberal or stringent than the Scheffe test? Provide a rationale for your answer.

4. Does the Bonferroni correction have a greater chance of a Type I or a Type II error than the Scheffe test? Provide a rationale for your answer.

5. The Bonferroni correction involves reducing the alpha as a basis for comparison with the study results. In this study, assume that 6 group comparisons were made. What was the alpha set at for the Bonferroni correction? Show your calculations.

6. Did Zampelas et al. (2005) note any differences in gender with regard to fish consumption and inflammatory markers? Discuss what this result means.

7. When compared with the non-fish consumers, those subjects who consumed > 300 g of fish per week had on average _____% lower CRP. Was this result significant? Provide a rationale for your answer.

8. What was the value of Amyloid A (mg/dl) for the group that made up the largest percentage of the sample? How much fish did this group consume?

9. Would the Tukey HSD test be a good choice as a post hoc analysis technique for this study? Provide a rationale for your answer.

10. Do the study findings have implications for health care? Provide a rationale for your answer.

ANALYSIS OF VARIANCE (ANOVA), CORRELATION COEFFICIENT, AND 95% CONFIDENCE INTERVAL

STATISTICAL TECHNIQUE IN REVIEW

The focus of this exercise is analysis of variance (ANOVA), correlation coefficients, and 95% confidence interval. ANOVA is conducted to examine differences between two or more groups and was discussed in Exercises 36 and 37. The outcome of ANOVA is a numerical value for the F statistic. A correlation coefficient (r) identifies the level of association between two variables and was the focus of Exercises 23 and 24. A confidence interval is represented by two numbers and is calculated with a 95% chance that the true study value falls somewhere between these two values and a 5% chance for error.

RESEARCH ARTICLE

Source: Agarwal, S., Allison, G. T., & Singer, K. P. (2005). Reliability of the spin-T cervical goniometer in measuring cervical range of motion in an asymptomatic Indian population. *Journal of Manipulative and Physiological Therapeutics, 28*(7), 487–92.

Introduction

The purpose of this study was to examine the reliability of the Spin-T, a cervical range of motion device, in a normal Indian population. "Subjects included 30 healthy adults with mean age of 34 years (range, 18–65 years). The subjects were stabilized in the sitting position the Spin-T goniometer mounted on the head[s]. . . . Three measurements were taken in each direction (flexion, extension lateral flexion, and lateral rotation) per participant. Reliability coefficients, intraclass correlation coefficients, and 95% confidence interval significances were derived from repeated measures analysis of variance (ANOVA). . . . In this study, the Spin-T goniometer proved to be a reliable measuring instrument for cervical range of movement in an Indian population" (Agarwal et al., 2005, p. 487). The subjects were recruited from the Belle Vue Clinic in Kolkata, India.

Relevant Study Results

The cervical movements were described with means and standard deviations. The intraclass correlation coefficient (ICC) values were high (> 0.96) for the six cervical movements, flexion, extension, lateral flexion (right and left), and lateral rotation (right and left) (see Table 2), thus, indicating that "the error was a small proportion of the total range of movement recorded" (Agarwal et al., 2005, p. 490.) The CIs for the correlational coefficients are also presented in Table 2. "The repeated-measures ANOVA (Table 3) showed no significant differences between the three trial measurements for flexion ($p = 0.17$), extension ($p = 0.12$), and lateral flexion (right $p = 0.65$, left $p = 0.45$)" (Agarwal et al., 2005, p. 490). The lateral rotation [both right and left] showed [a statistically significant difference between the three trial measurements] ($p < 0.01$)" (Agarwal et al., 2005, p. 490) (see Table 3). The level of statistical significance for this study was set at alpha (α) = 0.05. The findings from this study support the use of the Spin-T goniometer for measuring cervical range of motion in an Indian population. Additional research is needed to examine the reliability of this measurement device with larger samples and more diverse populations.

TABLE 2 ■ Intraobserver ICC Values and Their 95% CI for All Cervical Spine Movements

Movement	ICC	95% CI		F
		Lower	Upper	
Flexion	0.98	0.97	0.99	64.87
Extension	0.98	0.97	0.99	87.04
Lateral flexion(right)	0.96	0.93	0.98	27.72
Lateral flexion(left)	0.97	0.94	0.98	33.75
Lateral rotation(right)	0.98	0.97	0.99	71.89
Lateral rotation(left)	0.98	0.97	0.99	79.56

Agarwal, S., Allison, G. T., & Singer, K. P. (2005). Reliability of the spin-T cervical goniometer in measuring cervical range of motion in an asymptomatic Indian population. *Journal of Manipulative and Physiological Therapeutics, 28*(7), p. 489. Copyright © 2005, with permission from the National University of Health Sciences.

TABLE 3 ■ Repeated-Measures ANOVA to Measure Differences Between Trials for Movement in Each Direction

Movement	df	F	P
Flexion	2	1.79	.17
Extension	2	2.13	.12
Lateral flexion (right)	2	0.43	.65
Lateral flexion (left)	2	0.79	.45
Lateral rotation (right)	2	10.90	<.01
Lateral rotation (left)	2	13.44	<.01

Agarwal, S., Allison, G. T., & Singer, K. P. (2005). Reliability of the spin-T cervical goniometer in measuring cervical range of motion in an asymptomatic Indian population. *Journal of Manipulative and Physiological Therapeutics, 28*(7), p. 490. Copyright © 2005, with permission from the National University of Health Sciences.

■ STUDY QUESTIONS

1. According to Table 3, the *F* value for Lateral rotation (left) is 13.44. Is this result statistically significant? Provide a rationale for your answer.

2. According to Table 3, should the null hypothesis be rejected that there are no differences in the three trial measurements for Extension? Provide a rationale for your answer.

3. Table 3 displays non-significant F and p values for Lateral flexion right ($F = .43$, $p = 0.65$). What do these results mean?

4. What is the intraclass correlation coefficient (ICC) for Flexion? What does this value mean?

5. What are the values for the CI for Flexion in Table 2? Why is a CI calculated?

6. Table 3 displays F and p values for Lateral rotation (right). What do these results mean?

7. According to Table 2, do the ICC and the confidence intervals for Flexion and Extension have similarities? Provide a rationale for your answer.

8. What does the $df = 2$ mean in Table 3?

■ ANSWERS TO STUDY QUESTIONS

1. Yes, the $F = 13.44$ value for Lateral rotation (left) is statistically significant with $p < 0.01$. This p value is statistically significant because it is less than alpha set at 0.05.

2. No, the null hypothesis should not be rejected. The null hypothesis should be accepted since $F = 2.13$ is not statistically significant with $p = 0.12$, that is $> \alpha = 0.05$.

3. The results for Lateral flexion (right) indicate that there is no statistically significant difference in the three trial measurements of flexion with $p = 0.65$. The small differences between the three trial measurements are due to chance and not actual significant differences between the measurements.

4. The ICC = 0.98 for Flexion. This value indicates that there was reliability or consistency in the measurement of flexion and that the error was a small proportion of the total range of movement recorded.

5. The 95% CI for Flexion = 0.97 to 0.99. The CI produced has 95% chance of including the ICC for this study and a 5% chance of error.

6. The results for Lateral rotation right ($F = 10.90$, $p < 0.01$) indicate that there is a statistically significant difference among the three trial measurements for the right lateral rotation. This result of $p < 0.01$ is significant since it is less than alpha = 0.05.

7. Flexion ICC = 0.98 and 95% CI = 0.97 to 0.99. For Extension, ICC = 0.98 and 95% CI = 0.97 to 0.99. Yes, the measures for Extension and Flexion have the same reliability coefficient and 95% CI.

8. df stands for degrees of freedom for groups, and $df = 2$ since an ANOVA was conducted to determine differences between three trial measurements. The df for groups = $K - 1$. In this study, $K - 1 = 3 - 1 = 2$.

■ EXERCISE 39   Questions to be Graded

1. According to Table 2, no significant differences were found between the three trial measurements for which cervical movement? Provide a rationale for your answer.

2. According to Table 3, should the null hypothesis that there are no differences in the three trial measurements for Lateral Rotation (right) be rejected? Provide a rationale for your answer.

3. The ICC was lowest for which cervical range of motion measurement? What does this result indicate?

4. According to the article, a higher ICC value was obtained for same day measurements (ICC = 0.95) when compared to 1 to 3 days (ICC = 0.90). Although the ICC values were not statistically significantly different, what are some possibilities for the differences noted?

5. According to the study, all repeated measures showed high intraclass correlation coefficients (ICC) (all > 0.96, p =.01). What does this result mean?

6. Observing the *F* values in Table 2, can you determine whether these results were statistically significant or due to chance? Provide a rationale for your answer.

7. According to Table 2, we can be 95% sure that the ICC value for Extension falls between which two numbers? Provide a rationale for your answer.

8. A repeated-measures ANOVA was used in this study. Was this an appropriate analysis technique? Provide a rationale for your answer.

9. In Table 2, do the 95% confidence intervals overlap for the six cervical range of motion measurements? Why did this occur?

10. Are the findings from this study ready to be generalized to an Indian population? Provide a rationale for your answer.

CHI SQUARE (χ^2) I

STATISTICAL TECHNIQUE IN REVIEW

Chi Square (χ^2) is an inferential statistical test used to examine differences among groups with variables measured at the nominal level. χ^2 compares the frequencies that are observed with the frequencies that were expected. χ^2 calculations are compared with values in an χ^2 table. If the result is > or = ($\geq$) to the value in the table, significant differences exist. If values are statistically significant, the null hypothesis is rejected (Burns & Grove, *2005*). These results indicate that the differences are an actual reflection of reality and not due to random sampling error. If more than two groups are being examined, χ^2 does not determine where the differences lie; it only determines that a statistically significant difference exists. A post hoc analysis will determine the location of the difference. χ^2 is one of the weaker statistical tests used, and results are usually only reported if statistically significant values are found.

RESEARCH ARTICLE

Source: Salsberry, P. J. (2003). Why are some children still uninsured? *Journal of Pediatric Health Care,* *17*(1), 32–8.

Introduction

In an effort to understand why children remain uninsured, Salsberry (2003) interviewed low-income parents in Ohio and compared children with and without insurance. This cross-sectional survey design included a sample of 392 low-income parents. Subjects were chosen from two groups, those with a Medicaid history (*n* = 305) and those without a Medicaid history (*n* = 120). Those without a Medicaid history were chosen randomly. Results indicated specific profiles for different levels of insurance. These levels of insurance include uninsured, Medicaid-enrolled, and privately insured. "Statistically significant differences were found across the three groups in income, working status of the adults, education, health status of the adult and child, and in the utilization of health care" (Salsberry, 2003, p. 38). "Parents of the uninsured children were less knowledgeable about the application process. . . . Parents of uninsured children face multiple life challenges that may interfere with the enrollment process. Health problems, work schedules, and lack of knowledge may all need to be addressed before we can decrease the number of uninsured children in our nation" (Salsberry, 2003, p. 32).

Relevant Study Results

In Table 1, Salsberry (2003) presents the demographic characteristics of the sample by level of insurance (uninsured, Medicaid-enrolled, and privately insured).

TABLE 1 ■ Demographics of the Sample*				
	Uninsured (N = 62)	Medicaid (N = 219)	Privately Insured (N = 111)	χ^2
Gender–% female	34 (55%)	112 (51%)	55 (50%)	2.92
Race of child				
White	19 (31%)	80 (37%)	53 (48%)	6.45
African American	35 (56%)	118 (54%)	50 (45%)	
Other	8 (13%)	21 (10%)	8 (7%)	
Education (of adult)				
Less than 9	0	11 (5%)	1	24.60[‡]
10, 11, 12	14 (23%)	66 (30%)	15 (14%)	
High school grad	30 (48%)	83 (38%)	44 (40%)	
College or above	18 (29%)	59 (27%)	51 (46%)	
Marital status (%)				
Married/living with partner	18 (29%)	43 (20%)	49 (44%)	21.95[§]
Living alone	44 (71%)	176 (80%)	62 (56%)	
Working (%)				
Full/part-time	41 (66%)	104 (47%)	85 (77%)	27.39[§]
Not employed outside the home	21 (34%)	115 (53%)	26 (23%)	
No. in household				
2	8 (13%)	38 (17%)	11 (10%)	3.70
3	17 (27%)	51 (23%)	30 (27%)	
More than 3	37 (60%)	130 (60%)	70 (63%)	
Sample group				
Applied	39 (63%)	219 (100%)	51 (46%)	109.92[§]
Non-applied	23 (23%)	0	60 (54%)	
Adult health status				
Mean PCS	43.99	46.24	49.99	6.78[‡]
Mean MCS	48.03	47.56	50.11	1.84
Mean household income	$ 19,267	$ 16,833	$27,509	12.13[§]

*Not all cells add to the noted totals, because of missing data. Percents determined on valid responses.
Note: Adult health status and mean household income were compared using ANOVA.
[‡]$p \leq .05$.
[§]$p \leq .001$.
*($\leq$) = Less than or equal to the value
Working (%) varied among different levels of insurance. For example, in the Full/part-time group, 66% of parents were uninsured, 47% received Medicaid, and 77% were privately insured, [χ^2 (2,$N = 392$) = 27.39; $p = .001$].
In the Not employed outside the home group, 34% were uninsured, 53% received Medicaid, and 23% received private insurance.
Salsberry, P. J. (2003). Why are some children still uninsured? *Journal of Pediatric Health Care, 17*(1), p. 34, Copyright © 2003, with permission from The National Association of Pediatric Nurse Practitioners.

■ STUDY QUESTIONS

1. What was the sample size for this study?

2. What is the χ^2 value for Race of Child?

3. How many null hypotheses were accepted? Provide a rationale for your answer.

4. What is the χ^2 value for Marital Status (%): Married/living with partner or Living alone? Is the χ^2 value statistically significant? If significant, at what level?

5. The three groups (uninsured, Medicaid, and privately insured) are significantly different for the demographic variable Education (of adult) at $p \leq .05$. Are the groups also significantly different at $p \leq .001$? Provide a rationale for your answer.

6. Which has a greater statistically significant difference, Education (of adult) or Mean household income? Provide a rationale for your answer.

7. Mean household income is reported statistically significant at $p \leq .001$. Is it also statistically significant at $p \leq .05$? Provide a rationale for your answer.

8. State the null hypothesis for Mean household income and level of insurance (uninsured, Medicaid, and privately insured).

9. Should the null hypothesis for Question 8 be accepted or rejected? Provide a rationale for your answer.

10. In your opinion, when compared to level of insurance, what do the values reported for Working (%): Full/part-time and Not employed outside the home mean? Provide a rationale for your answer.

■ ANSWERS TO STUDY QUESTIONS

1. The sample size was 392 ($N = 392$) as indicated in the "Introduction."
2. In Table 1, the $\chi^2 = 6.45$ for the Race of Child.
3. Four null hypotheses were accepted since four χ^2 values were not significant, as indicated in Table 1. Nonsignificant results indicate that the null hypotheses are supported or accepted as an accurate reflection of the results of the study.
4. The $\chi^2 = 21.95$ for Marital Status (%): Married/living with partner or Living alone. The symbol next to this χ^2 value indicates that it is statistically significant at $p \le .001$. If alpha (α) $= 0.05$ for this study, then p is less than α indicates that the χ^2 value is statistically significant.
5. No, $p \le .001$ has a greater significance than $p \le .05$, since the smaller the p value, the more significant the findings. Thus, $p \le .05$ is not as significant as at $p \le .001$.
6. Mean household income has a greater statistically significant value because it is reported significant at $p \le .001$, whereas Education (of adult) is reported significant at $p \le .05$. The smaller the p value, the more significant the findings.
7. Yes, Mean household income is also significant at $p \le .05$, since $p \le .001$ has a greater significance than $p \le .05$. What is significant at $p \le .001$ is also significant at $p \le .05$.
8. There is no difference in Mean household income among the three groups determined by levels of insurance (uninsured, Medicaid-enrolled, and privately insured).
9. The null hypothesis should be rejected. Mean household income is reported statistically significant at $p \le .001$. Thus, the null hypothesis is rejected when statistical significance is found.
10. Answers may vary. As parents begin to work either full- or part-time and earn a paycheck, the chances that they will be able to qualify for Medicaid decrease, whereas the ability for them to afford private insurance may not always increase. Often parents will make enough money to disqualify them for Medicaid but not enough money to afford private insurance. This is one explanation for a higher uninsured percentage, a lower Medicaid percentage, and a higher private insurance percentage than the Not employed outside the home group reported in Table 1.

■ EXERCISE 40   Questions to be Graded

1. According to the "Introduction," what categories were reported to be statistically significant?

2. In Table 1, is the No. in household reported as statistically significant among the three groups (uninsured, Medicaid, and privately insured)? Provide a rationale for your answer.

3. Should the null hypothesis for Marital Status (%) be rejected? Provide a rationale for your answer.

4. How many null hypotheses were rejected in the Salsberry (2003) study? Provide a rationale for your answer.

5. Does Marital Status or Education (of adults) have a greater statistically significant difference among the three groups (uninsured, Medicaid, or privately insured)? Provide a rationale for your answer.

6. Was there a significant difference in Working status for the three levels of insurance (uninsured, Medicaid-enrolled, and privately insured)? Provide a rationale for your answer.

7. State the null hypothesis for level of insurance and Gender–% female.

8. Should the null hypothesis for Question 7 be accepted or rejected? Provide a rationale for your answer.

9. In your own opinion, were the outcomes of this study what you expected?

10. In your own opinion, should the results of this study be generalized to other State Children's Health Insurance Programs (SCHIPs)? Provide a rationale for your answer.

41

CHI SQUARE (χ^2) II

STATISTICAL TECHNIQUE IN REVIEW

The introduction to the chi square (χ^2) analysis technique is provided in Exercise 40. In addition to the χ^2 value, researchers often report the degrees of freedom (df). This mathematically complex statistical concept is important for calculating and determining levels of significance. The standard formula for df is: sample size (N) minus 1 or $df = N - 1$ (Burns & Grove, 2005); however, this formula is adjusted based on the analysis technique performed. The formula for df for χ^2 is: $df = (R - 1)(C - 1)$, where R is number of rows and C is the number of columns in a chi square table. For example, in a 3 x 2 chi square table $df = (3 - 1)(2 - 1) = 2$. In the following example, df is presented in the ( ): $\chi^2 (2, N = 392) = 21.95$; $p < .0001$. Therefore, the df is equal to 2. It is important to note that the df can also be reported without the sample size, as in $\chi^2_{(2)}$. For additional information regarding χ^2, please refer to Exercise 40.

RESEARCH ARTICLE

Source: Brewer, C. S., & Nauenberg, E. (2003). Future intentions of registered nurses employed in the western New York labor market: Relationships among demographic, economic, and attitudinal factors. *Applied Nursing Research*, *16*(3), 144–55.

Introduction

In an effort to determine if demographic, economic, and attitudinal factors influence workplace participation or cause registered nurses (RNs) to leave their current job position, Brewer and Nauenberg (2003) reviewed surveys of RNs working in western New York. The sample consisted of 776 randomly selected RNs under the age of 65. Full and part-time RNs working in hospital and non-hospital settings were examined and tested for differences with classical *t*-tests and chi square tests. For the purposes of this study, economic factors include wages, benefits, and collective bargaining; and attitudinal factors include satisfaction, organizational commitment, and job perceptions. The researchers found that only "RNs employed in hospital settings were significantly less satisfied and less committed to their organization than were non-hospital based nurses; however these attitudes, frequently shown to be related to turnover behavior, did not result in intentions to leave. Differences in satisfaction and commitment across job settings begin to explain work participation behavior of nurses, as distinct from organizational behavior" (Brewer & Nauenberg, 2003, p. 144). This study is important because it connects the idea of job satisfaction and organizational commitment across different job settings.

Relevant Study Results

Important demographic information reported in the research article include 97.3% of the sample group was Caucasian, 41.7% of the sample group held an associate's degree, and only a 0.8% of the RNs were under the age of 30. "Hospital and part-time RNs were younger than the hospital/full-time RNs and had 2 to 3 years less experience than their counterparts. . . . Women are significantly more likely to work part-time than are men, and hospital-based workers were more likely to be unionized than were non-hospital workers. There were no significant differences by race, multiple jobs, or children's age" (Brewer & Nauenberg, 2003, p. 146). The researchers reported a survey response rate of 54.1% for their study. For this exercise, Table 1 has been adjusted to include only the chi square tests.

TABLE 1 ■ Significant Demographic Factors: Age, Work Experience, Weeks Worked, Gender, Children, Union Representation, Marital Status, Spousal Work Status

Total Sample Statistic	FT/PT STATUS BY WORK VENUE					WORK VENUE		FT/PT STATUS			
	Grand Mean *(SD)* n=776	Hospital FT *(SD)* n=232	Non-hospital FT *(SD)* n=208	Hospital PT *(SD)* n=113	Non-hospital PT *(SD)* n=108	Hospital *(SD)* n=345	Non-hospital *(SD)* n=318	FT *(SD)* n=442	PT *(SD)* n=221	Not Working *(SD)* n=113	
Education (%)											
• Diploma	26.9	28	22.6	23.9	30.6	27.1	25.6	25.7	27.6	30	$\chi^2(3) = 13.5**$
† AD	41.7	45.3	38.9	38.9	37	43.8	42.2	42.9	41.9	36.4	$\chi^2(3) = 3.24$
‡ BA/BS	29.8	24.6	32.7	36.3	32.4	28.8	30	28.9	30.4	31.8	$\chi^2(3) = 4.97$
§MA or higher	1.7	.4	4.8	0	1.9	.3	3.2	2.5	0	1.8	$\chi^2(3) = 3.89$
Sample size for Spousal work status	n=585	n=164	n=144	n=98	n=89	n=262	n=234	n=309	n=187	n=89	
• Spousal work status	82.2	82.3	83.3	91.8	85.4	85.9	84.2	82.8	88.8	66.3	$\chi^2(2) = 1.08$
† Spouse works FT (%)											$\chi^2(2) = 2.02$
‡ Spousal works PT (%)	7.2	8.5	10.4	3.1	4.5	6.5	8.1	9.4	3.7	6.7	$\chi^2(2) = 0.48$ $\chi^2(2) = 5.73*$

The chi square (χ^2) test was used to test for differences across the multiple work intention categories.
• Hospital full-time/non-hospital full-time comparison
† Hospital part-time/non-hospital part-time comparison
‡ Hospital/non-hospital comparison
§ Full-time/part-time comparison
* $p \le 0.05$
** $p \le 0.01$

Brewer, C. S., & Nauenberg, E. (2003). Future intentions of registered nurses employed in the western New York labor market: Relationships among demographic, economic, and attitudinal factors. *Applied Nursing Research, 16*(3), p. 147.

■ STUDY QUESTIONS

1. Of the χ^2 results reported in Table 1, how many were statistically significant? Provide a rationale for your answer.

2. State the null hypothesis for Education (%): MA or higher variable found in Table 1.

3. What is the χ^2 value for Education (%): MA or higher when comparing full-time and part-time work status groups? Is the χ^2 value statistically significant? If the value is statistically significant, at what level?

4. Based on the answers to Questions 2 and 3, should the null hypotheses be accepted or rejected? Provide a rationale for your answer.

5. In Table 1, is the value for Education (%): BA/BS when hospital and non-hospital groups are compared statistically significant? Provide a rationale for your answer.

6. In Table 1, Spousal work status is compared between hospital full-time and non-hospital full-time groups. What does the (2) represent in χ^2 (2) = 1.08?

7. In Table 1, the χ^2 = 13.5** has a footnote, which indicates that it is significant at $p \leq 0.01$. Using a statistics book, look up $p < 0.01$ with 2 degrees of freedom in a table of X^2 critical values. What must the value be to yield statistical significance?

8. Table 1 lists the value of * $p \leq 0.05$. What does this value mean? Provide a rationale for your answer.

9. Based on the information provided in Table 1, what 4 pairs of groups are the χ^2 tests being calculated to compare?

10. Which group was the largest? Which group was the smallest? Are these results surprising? Provide a rationale for your answer.

ANSWERS TO STUDY QUESTIONS

1. In Table 1, the results from eight χ^2 tests were reported and only two of the χ^2 values were statistically significant as indicated by the table key of the significant p values, $*p \leq 0.05$ and $**p \leq 0.01$. One χ^2 test, Education (%): Diploma, was reported to be statistically significant at $p \leq 0.01$, and Spousal works PT (%) for the hospital/non-hospital comparison was statistically significant at $p \leq 0.05$.

2. There is no difference for Education (%): MA or higher when full-time and part-time work status groups are compared.

3. The $\chi^2 = 3.89$ when full-time and part-time groups are compared for Education (%): MA or higher. This χ^2 value is not statistically significant at either $p \leq 0.05$ or $p \leq 0.01$ since there is no * after the value.

4. The null hypotheses for Question 2 should be accepted. If the χ^2 value is not statistically significant, then the null hypothesis should be accepted. The $\chi^2 = 3.89$ is not statistically significant.

5. In Table 1, the $\chi^2 = 4.97$ for Education (%): BA/BS when compared between hospital and non-hospital groups. This value is not statistically significant at either $p \leq 0.05$ or $p \leq 0.01$ since the χ^2 value has no * next to it that is used to identify significant findings in this study.

6. In Table 1, the (2) in χ^2 (2) = 1.08 represents the degrees of freedom (*df*) for Spousal work status compared between the hospital full-time and non-hospital full-time groups.

7. Using a table of χ^2 Critical Values from a statistical or research textbook (Burns & Grove, 2005, p. 707), with 2 *df* at $p \leq 0.01$, the χ^2 value must be ≥ 9.21 to be significant. Values might vary slightly based on the table you are using.

8. The symbol p stands for probability and $\leq$ is synonymous with the phrase less than or equal to. The value $* p \leq 0.05$ indicates the significance of the χ^2 values in Table 1. Only $\chi^2 = 5.73*$ is significant at $p \leq 0.05$.

9. Based on the information found in Table 1, the 4 pairs of groups being compared with the χ^2 tests include:
Hospital full-time/non-hospital full-time comparison ($\bullet$)
Hospital part-time/non-hospital part-time comparison (†)
Hospital/non-hospital comparison (‡)
Full-time/part-time comparison (§)

10. The largest group was full-time hospital RNs with $n = 232$ and the smallest group was non-hospital part-time RNs with $n = 108$. Rationale for answers may vary. No, these results are not surprising, since most nurses do work a full-time job and often in the hospital. Many RNs like the flexibility of hospital scheduling, with the 12-hour shifts and the 36-hour work week. Also, the majority of nursing jobs are in the hospital. Non-hospital jobs may provide less compensation and flexibility. The demand for non-hospital nursing is not as high as hospital nursing. Non-hospital jobs may require more experience, which is a deterrent to new practicing RNs.

Name: _____ _____ Class: _____

Date: _____

■ EXERCISE 41   Questions to be Graded

1. Examine the χ^2 values reported in Table 1. Are any of the values reported statistically significant at $p \leq 0.05$?

2. State the null hypothesis for Spouse works PT (%) in comparison with the hospital and non-hospital groups. Should the null hypothesis be accepted or rejected? Provide a rationale for your answer.

3. In Table 1, Education (%): BA/BS, is compared between hospital and non-hospital groups. What does the (3) represent in χ^2 (3) = 4.97?

4. For this research article, *df* was reported. However, in Exercise 40, *df* was not reported. In your opinion, should *df* be reported? Provide a rationale for your answer.

5. What is the χ^2 value reported for Education (%): AD when comparing the hospital part-time and non-hospital part-time groups of RNs? Is this χ^2 value significant? Provide a rationale for your answer.

6. Table 1 lists the value of ** $p \leq 0.01$. What does this value mean?

7. Using the information from Question 5 and a χ^2 Critical Value Table, look up the χ^2 value for Education (%): AD at $p \leq 0.05$ and $p \leq 0.01$ at 3 df. What are these two values, and do they support the finding being non-significant?

8. Review the χ^2 values in the χ^2 Critical Values Table of a research or statistical textbook. What conclusions can you draw about the χ^2 values and the level of significance of these values in the table?

9. Brewer and Nauenberg (2003) concluded that only "Only RNs employed in hospital settings were significantly less satisfied and less committed to their organization than were non-hospital based nurses; however, these attitudes, frequently shown to be related to turnover behavior, did not result in intentions to leave" (Brewer & Nauenberg, 2003, p. 144). Discuss the meaning of this finding, and provide a rationale for this finding.

10. In your own opinion, should the results of this study be generalized to other nursing populations in other states? Provide a rationale for your answer.

42

SPEARMAN RANK-ORDER CORRELATION COEFFICIENT

STATISTICAL TECHNIQUE IN REVIEW

The **Spearman Rank-Order Correlation Coefficient,** or **Spearman *rho*,** is a nonparametric test used to identify relationships between two variables. The Spearman analysis technique is an adaptation of the Pearson Product-Moment Correlation (see Exercises 23 and 24) and is used when the assumptions of the Pearson's analysis cannot be met. Thus, the Spearman *rho* analysis technique is used to analyze data that are ordinal level of measurement or scores measured at the interval or ratio levels that are skewed or not normally distributed. Scores must be ranked to conduct this analysis. Each subject included in the analysis must have a score (or value) on each of two variables, variable *x* and variable *y*. The scores on each variable are ranked separately (Burns & Grove, 2005).

Calculation of Spearmen *rho* is based on **difference scores** between a subject's ranking on the first (variable *x*) and second (variable *y*) sets of scores. The formula for difference scores is $D = x - y$. Since results with negative scores cancel out positive scores, results are squared for use in the analysis. The formula for calculation of Spearman *rho* is:

$$rho = 1 - \frac{6\sum D^2}{N^3 - N}$$

Where:
rho = Statistic for the Spearman correlation coefficient
D = Difference between the rankings of a subject's score on both variables *x* and *y*
N = Number of paired ranked scores

The Spearman Rank-Order Correlation Coefficient values range from –1 to +1, where a positive number indicates a positive relationship and a negative number indicates a negative relationship. Numbers closest to +1 or −1 indicate the strongest relationships. In comparison to the linear correlation coefficient, Spearman *rho* has an efficiency of 91% in detecting an existing relationship. The strength of *rho* values are: < 0.3 or < −0.3 are weak relationships, 0.3 to 0.5 or −0.3 to −0.5 are moderate relationships, and > 0.5 or > −0.5 are strong relationships.

Spearman *rho* is calculated using the following hypothetical example, where five students' intramuscular (IM) injection techniques were ranked by two instructors from a high score of 1 to a low score of 5. The purpose is to see if there is a relationship between the two instructors' rankings of the 5 students' IM injection techniques.

Student	Instructor A	Instructor B	D	D²
Amy	1	3	–2	4
Jeff	3	2	1	1
John	5	4	1	1
Julie	2	1	1	1
Mary	4	5	–1	1
Sum				8

Calculations:

$$rho = 1 - \frac{6\sum D^2}{N^3 - N} \qquad rho = 1 - \frac{6(8)}{125 - 5} = 1 - \frac{48}{120} = 1 - 0.4 = 0.6$$

In this example, a strong positive correlation or relationship ($rho = 0.6$) was found between the two instructors' ranking of students on IM injection techniques.

RESEARCH ARTICLE

Source: Kugler, C., Vlaminck, H., Haverich, A., & Maes, B., (2005). Nonadherence with diet and fluid restrictions among adults having hemodialysis. *Journal of Nursing Scholarship, 37*(1), 25–29.

Introduction

A multicenter cross-sectional study design was used to measure nonadherence of prescribed diet and fluid restrictions among patients receiving hemodialysis. The sample included 916 patients. The patients were chosen from dialysis centers using a convenience sampling method when the centers "met the following inclusion criteria: size of more than 50 hospital-based or outpatient dialysis patients; willingness to include all eligible patients; and giving written informed consent" (Kugler et al., 2005, p. 26). Eligible patients were asked to complete the Dialysis Diet and Fluid Nonadherence Questionnaire (DDFQ). "Nonadherence was measured by asking frequency and intensity of deviation from diet and fluid restrictions during the previous 14 days" (Kugler et al., 2005, p. 26). "Biological and biochemical lab values were collected from medical records in the presence of the patients. . . . The sample included 484 (52.9%) male and 432 (47.1%) female patients from 19 to 91 years (median 67). The average time on dialysis was 47 months with a range from 3 months to 28 years" (Kugler et al., 2005, p. 26).

"The results showed that many patients had difficulty following diet (81.4%) and fluid (74.6%) restrictions. Younger male patients and smokers were at highest risk for nonadherence. Higher levels of interdialysis weight gain were associated with nonadherence. . . . The findings indicate the need to continue to monitor and study hemodialysis patients' adherence behavior longitudinally and to design interventions to enhance adherence" (Kugler et al., 2005, p. 25).

Relevant Study Results

Frequency and degree of nonadherence to diet and fluid restrictions were correlated with the biochemical values with Spearman *rho* coefficients. The frequency of diet nonadherence correlated positively with the IWG [interdialysis weight gain] ($p = 0.0001$), albumin ($p = 0.0001$), and phosphate ($p = 0.002$). For the frequency of fluid nonadherence, positive correlations were found for IWG ($p = 0.0001$), phosphate ($p = 0.0001$), potassium ($p = 0.013$), and albumin ($p = 0.015$)" (Kugler et al., 2005, p. 27). The results of the Spearman Rank-Order Correlation analysis are shown in Table 2 and the level of significance for this study was set at α 0.05.

"The results also showed a strong correlation between frequency and degree of fluid nonadherence ($p = 0.0001$), and between the frequency of diet and fluid nonadherence ($p = 0.0001$)" (Kugler et al., 2005, p. 27). Weak, positive correlations were identified for the other variables (see Table 3). The *r* in Tables 2 and 3 is used to represent the results of Spearman Rank-Order Correlation coefficient that would have been more accurately presented with *rho* as the statistic.

"Nonadherence was also calculated in relation to the demographic variables, smoking, and comorbidities. Male gender was associated with frequency and degree (diet and fluid) of nonadherence ($p = 0.0001$). Young age was correlated with diet and fluid nonadherence ($p = 0.001$). A significant correlation was found for social support and the frequency of fluid nonadherence ($p = 0.005$), but not for diet nonadherence" (Kugler et al., 2005, pp. 27–8).

Strong relationships were found between "smoking and frequency and intensity of nonadherence to both diet and fluid restrictions ($p = 0.0001$). Time on dialysis showed a positive significant correlation to the degree of nonadherence ($p = 0.015$, diet; $p = 0.003$, fluid), but not for frequency of nonadherence" (Kugler et al., 2005, p. 28).

TABLE 2 ■ Correlation of Nonadherence With Biochemical and Biological Variables

	Potassium r(p)	Phosphate r(p)	Albumin r(p)	IWG r(p)
Frequency of diet nonadherence	ns	.104 (.002)	.221 (.0001)	.226 (.0001)
Degree of diet nonadherence	.109 (.001)	.072 (.030)	.206 (.0001)	.258 (.0001)
Frequency of fluid nonadherence	.082 (.013)	.120 (.0001)	.109 (.015)	.349 (.0001)
Degree of fluid nonadherence	.092 (.005)	.099 (.003)	.180 (.0001)	.351 (.0001)

Kugler, C., Vlaminck, H., Haverich, A., & Maes, B., (2005). Nonadherence with diet and fluid restrictions among adults having hemodialysis. *Journal of Nursing Scholarship, 37*(1), p. 27.

TABLE 3 ■ Correlation Matrix for Frequency and Degree of Nonadherence Regarding Diet and Fluid (r[p])

	Frequency diet	Degree diet	Frequency fluid	Degree fluid
Frequency diet		.650 (.0001)	.502 (.0001)	.385 (.0001)
Degree diet			.398 (.0001)	.484 (.0001)
Frequency fluid				.750 (.0001)
Degree fluid				

Kugler, C., Vlaminck, H., Haverich, A., & Maes, B., (2005). Nonadherence with diet and fluid restrictions among adults having hemodialysis. *Journal of Nursing Scholarship, 37*(1), p. 28.

"This study was limited by the design with only one measurement point. No evidence was ascertained about patients' adherence over time. Furthermore, limitations might have pertained to cultural preferences regarding eating and drinking patterns in only two European areas [Belgium and Germany]. Finally, adherence is difficult to assess objectively. The validity of the patients' responses may have been influenced by their desire to present themselves in the best possible light, which could have confounded the findings of the study. . . . Because of the life-long duration of the treatment, strategies to improve adherence, such as patient education programs, and strategies to maintain and reactivate adherence, such as regular educational follow-up, are indicated" (Kugler et al., 2005, p. 28–9).

■ STUDY QUESTIONS

1. What is the relationship between frequency of diet nonadherence and albumin?

2. Is there a relationship between degree of diet nonadherence and potassium? Provide a rationale for your answer.

3. Describe the relationship between degree of diet nonadherence and albumin. What is the strength of this relationship, is it positive or negative, and is it statistically significant? Provide rationales for your answers.

4. What do the results *r* or *rho* = 0.351, *p* = 0.0001 mean? Discuss what this result means for the patient.

5. What was the weakest relationship presented in Table 2? Was this relationship statistically significant? Provide a rationale for your answer.

6. Is there a stronger correlation between frequency of fluid nonadherence and albumin or degree of fluid nonadherence and albumin? Provide a rationale for your answer.

7. Describe the relationship between degree of diet nonadherence and IWG (interdialysis weight gain).

8. What do the results for Question 7 mean, and what is the influence on the patient?

9. Why was the Spearman Rank-Order Correlation Coefficient used to examine the relationships in this study?

ANSWERS TO STUDY QUESTIONS

1. Frequency of diet nonadherence is related to albumin with $r = 0.221$.

2. Yes, there is a relationship between degree of diet nonadherence and potassium as indicated by r or $rho = 0.109$. This is a weak, positive relationship between these two variables.

3. The relationship between degree of diet nonadherence and albumin is r or $rho = 0.206$ ($p = 0.0001$). This is a weak, positive relationship that is statistically significant at $p = 0.0001$, which is smaller than alpha that was set at 0.05. If a p value is less than alpha, then the result is statistically significant.

4. r or $rho = 0.351$, $p = 0.0001$, means that degree of fluid nonadherence has a moderate, positive relationship with IWG. This relationship is statistically significant, which means that patients with greater weight gains are also likely to be patients with greater levels of nonadherence to their fluid restrictions. Thus, these patients are likely to have more health problems than patients who comply with their fluid restrictions.

5. The weakest relationship was between frequency of diet nonadherence and potassium. This was a nonsignificant (*ns*) relationship and no value was provided. Researchers often do not present the specific results for nonsignificant findings.

6. The stronger correlation is between degree of fluid nonadherence and albumin with r or $rho = 0.180$ ($p = 0.0001$). The relationship between frequency of fluid nonadherence and albumin is weaker with r or $rho = 0.109$ ($p = 0.015$), which is < 0.180. The $p = 0.015$ is larger than the $p = 0.0001$, which indicates that the relationship between degree of fluid nonadherence and albumin is the most significant. The smaller the p value, the more significant the results are in a study.

7. The relationship between degree of diet nonadherence and IWG is positive, weak, and significant with $r = 0.258$ ($p = 0.0001$). Thus, as the degree of diet nonadherence increases so does the IWG.

8. The results in Question 7 indicate that as a patient's degree of diet nonadherence worsens so does their interdialysis weight gain. Thus, patients who do not follow their diet restrictions have greater weight gain and more potential for health problems.

9. The Spearman *rho* was used to examine the relationships in this study since the variables of frequency of diet nonadherence, degree of diet nonadherence, frequency of fluid nonadherence, and degree of fluid nonadherence were measured at the ordinal level. These variables were measured with the DDFQ, and the subjects were rank-ordered based on their scores on the DDFQ.

■ EXERCISE 42   Questions to be Graded

1. Identify the variables in Table 3. Are the relationships among these variables positive or negative? Provide a rationale for your answer.

2. What two variables from Table 3 have the strongest positive correlation? Provide a rationale for your answer.

3. What do the results in Question 2 mean? How might this information be used in educating patients on dialysis?

4. According to the study narrative, a strong, positive correlation exists between frequency and degree of diet nonadherence. How can this be verified using Table 3?

5. According to the Relevant Study Results, young age correlated with diet and fluid nonadherence ($p = 0.001$). Assuming the correlation is negative, what do these results mean? How might health care providers use this information in managing young patients on hemodialysis?

6. Describe the relationship between frequency of fluid nonadherence and IWG. Discuss how this result might be used in practice.

7. According to the Relevant Study Results, how was the degree of nonadherence related to time on dialysis? How might this information be used in practice?

8. Identify some of the limitations of this study. How would these limitations impact the study findings?

9. The Kugler et al. (2005) study results include moderate to strong positive correlations between frequency and degree of nonadherence behaviors for diet and fluid restrictions. Assuming that these study findings were ready to generalize to all hemodialysis patients, what are some of the possible implications for nursing practice?

10. Calculate the Spearman *rho* value for the evaluations of four nurses' patient care by two managers, with 1 indicating the highest quality of care and 4 indicating the lowest quality of care.

Nurses	Manager #1 Rankings	Manager #2 Rankings
M. Jones	3	4
C. Smith	2	3
T. Robert	1	1
S. Hart	4	2

43

MANN-WHITNEY U TEST

STATISTICAL TECHNIQUE IN REVIEW

Mann-Whitney U test is a nonparametric analysis technique used to detect differences between two independent groups. The Mann-Whitney U test is the most powerful of the nonparametric tests, with 95% of the power of the t-test. If the assumptions for the t-test cannot be satisfied, that is, if ordinal-level data are collected or the distribution of scores is skewed or not normal, then the Mann-Whitney U is the analysis technique of choice. To calculate the value of U, scores of both groups are combined and each score is assigned a rank. The lowest score is ranked 1, the next score is ranked 2, and so forth until all scores are ranked, regardless of which group the score was from. The idea is that if two distributions came from the same population, the average of the ranks of their scores would be equal as well (Burns & Grove, 2005).

RESEARCH ARTICLE

Source: Tsai, S. L. (2003). The effects of a research utilization in-service program on nurses. *International Journal of Nursing Studies, 40*(2), 105–13.

Introduction

Tsai (2003) conducted a quasi-experimental study to examine the impact of an 8-week research utilization course on nurses' attitudes towards nursing research, their research participation, and utilization of research findings. Study participants were divided into an experimental group ($n = 47$) and a control group ($n = 42$); a pretest (T1), posttest (T2), and a 6-month follow-up (T3) tests were administered. To evaluate the nurses' attitudes towards research, a 29-item scale with a 5-point scoring system, where 5 meant total agreement and 1 meant total disagreement, was developed. Higher scores denoted more positive attitudes towards nursing research. The researchers used t-tests to compare test scores of both groups. The experimental group displayed a more positive attitude towards research than the control group.

The Mann-Whitney U test was used to measure the differences in research participation between the experimental and the control groups over time. Subjects' scores were calculated using a 33-item questionnaire with a 2-point scoring system, where 1 meant participation in a particular activity and 0 meant no participation. The alpha or the level of significance for this study was set at 0.05. "The results showed that there were significant differences in attitudes between the two groups toward research and perceived support of institutions. Participation in research also differed significantly when analyzed at posttests 2 and 6 months after the course. There was no significant difference in research utilization. These results suggest that continuous consultation and assistance should be provided to the nurses after the course, so as to implement the results of research utilization" (Tsai, 2003, p. 105).

Relevant Study Results

"The degree of research participation was compared between the two groups by the Mann-Whitney *U* test. There were no significant differences between the two groups in the pretest comparison ($z = -0.7$, $p > 0.05$)" (Tsai, 2003, p. 109). However, the differences were significant at T2 ($z = -3.75$, $p < 0.05$) and at T3 ($z = -2.96$, $p < 0.05$) after the research utilization courses. Nurses in the experimental group had a higher degree of research participation [during the study than those in the control group] (Table 3).

TABLE 3 ■ Research Participation Over Time (*N=89*)			MANN–WHITNEY *U*	
Variables	*n*	Median (0–33)	*z*	*p*
Pretest			−0.07	0.944
Control	42	5.80		
Experimental	47	6.00		
T2			−3.75	0.000
Control	42	4.00		
Experimental	47	8.00		
T3			−2.96	0.003
Control	42	4.50		
Experimental	47	9.00		

Note: T2—at the completion of the course; T3—6 month after completion of the course.
Tsai, S. L. (2003). The effects of a research utilization in-service program on nurses. *International Journal of Nursing Studies, 40*(2), p. 110.

■ STUDY QUESTIONS

1. One of the research hypotheses from this study was: "Nurses who attend the research utilization course have higher score of participation in nursing research than those who do not" (Tsai, 2003, p. 106). State the null hypothesis.

2. What does "(0–33)" after the word "median" represent?

3. Mann-Whitney *U* is the appropriate statistical test to use in which of the following situations:
   a. Interval/ratio level data with a skewed distribution of scores for study variables.
   b. The difference between two dependent groups is being examined.
   c. The data collected are at the nominal level of measurement.
   d. Correlation or relationship between two groups is being examined.

4. Why were the medians versus means selected as the measure of central tendency for describing the variables in this study?

5. Was there a statistically significant difference between the control and the experimental groups at the 6-month follow-up test (T3)? Provide a rationale for your answer.

6. The researchers analyzed the nurses' attitude data as though it were at what level of measurement?
   a. Nominal
   b. Ordinal
   c. Interval/ratio
   d. Abstract

7. If the researchers decided to compare the nurses' attitude posttest scores (T2) of the experimental group to its 6-month follow-up (T3) scores, what test would they have used? Provide a rationale for your answer.
   a. Mann-Whitney *U* test
   b. *t*-test for independent samples
   c. Chi-squared (χ^2)
   d. *t*-test for dependent samples.

8. Compare the median values of the experimental and the control groups over time. What trends do you note in the research participation in both of these groups? How might this affect the significant differences between these two groups?

■ ANSWERS TO STUDY QUESTIONS

1. The null hypothesis is: There is no difference between the nursing research participation of nurses who attend a research utilization course and those who do not.

2. "(0–33)" represents the range of all possible scores of subjects for participation in research as measured by a questionnaire in this study. The questionnaire had 33 items, and a score of 1 meant participation in the research activity and the 0 meant no participation. Thus, subjects who did not participate in research would have a low score closer to 0 and those actively participating in a research would have a score closer to 33. This questionnaire produces data that are at the ordinal level. The scores of the nurses can be rank-ordered for their level of participation in research activities.

3. a. Interval/ratio level data with a skewed distribution of scores for study variables. Since it is a nonparametric test, the Mann-Whitney *U* test should be used for interval/ratio level data when the requirements for using a parametric test cannot be satisfied, that is, when the collected data has a skewed or non-normal distribution. The Mann-Whitney *U* test is to be used with independent and not dependent or related groups and is for at least ordinal level data and not nominal level data. The Mann-Whitney *U* test is designed to determine differences and not test for relationships.

4. The research participation questionnaire produced ordinal level data. When data collected are at the ordinal level of measurement, the median is the most accurate measure of central tendency to analyze such data (Burns & Grove, 2007). The median is also the most accurate measure of central tendency for interval/ratio data that is skewed. The mean should only be calculated for normally distributed interval/ratio data.

5. $p = 0.003$ at the 6-month follow-up test (T3), which indicates the result is statistically significant since the p value is less than alpha that was set at 0.05 for this study.

6. c. Interval/ratio. The researchers used *t*-tests to detect differences in nurses' attitudes between the experimental and the control groups. The *t*-test is a parametric test for differences used when analyzing data from study variables measured at the interval or ratio level. Even though their attitudes were measured using an ordinal 5-point scoring scale, the researchers used the total score of the scale for each participant, that is, summed up all of his/her attitude scores for each of the 29 items of the scale, and considered the data at the interval/ratio level of measurement (Burns & Grove, 2005).

7. d. *t*-test for dependent samples. The researchers would have used a *t*-test for dependent groups since the test scores of the same group (the experimental group) are being compared at two different times, at the completion of the course and 6 months after completion of the course. The Mann-Whitney *U* test and *t*-test for independent groups can only be used when analyzing data obtained from independent groups. The Chi-square test is utilized when nominal level data are being analyzed.

8. The experimental median values increased over time, indicating that research participation was increasing in this group; the median values for the control group decreased, indicating decreased research participation. The significant differences in posttest results between the two groups were observed not only because the median scores of the experimental group were higher after the research utilization in-service program but also because the scores of the control group were lower on both posttests. Had the latter phenomenon not occurred, the differences between the two groups would have still been significant but probably not as significant. The declining participation score of the control group is an example of a phenomenon called "regression towards the true mean." This occurs when repeated measurements are obtained over time, and subjects' scores are likely to become more reflective of the true level of attribute they possess. In this study, the control group participants probably scored higher on the pretest simply because of the awareness that their research participation was being studied. As time passed, the control group participants got used to the idea that research was being conducted and their scores decreased, reflecting the true amount of research participation activities of these subjects.

■ EXERCISE 43   Questions to be Graded

1. What was the total number of the research participants for this study?

2. In Table 3, which p values are significant and which are not?

3. Why was the Mann-Whitney U test and not the t-test used to examine the differences in research participation between the two groups?

4. In Table 3, what comparison demonstrated the greatest significant difference between the groups? Provide a rationale for your answer.

5. Does the p value of the pretest enhance or diminish the validity of the findings? Provide a rationale for your answer.

6. What might have been the reason why the researchers did not treat the participation questionnaire data as interval data (by using the subjects' total scores on the questionnaire) and conducted *t*-tests instead of the Mann-Whitney *U* test as they did when nurses' attitudes towards research were examined? (Hint: Look at the median scores and compare them to the range.)

7. If the researcher ran a skewness analysis on the distribution of scores presented in Table 3 and found that the distribution was skewed, would the data be positively or negatively skewed? Would the direction of skewness be a positive or negative outcome for this study? Provide a rationale for your answer. If needed, review Exercise 19, "Determining Skewness of a Distribution."

8. According to Table 3, did the research utilization in-service program have a lasting effect on the research participation activities scores of the members of the experimental group? Provide a rationale for your answer.

9. The *p* value for the posttest (T2) equals 0.000. What does this result mean?

10. Could researchers use the Mann-Whitney *U* test to compare the performance of the experimental group between the pretest and the posttest? Provide a rationale for your answer.

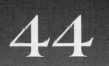

44 WILCOXON MATCHED-PAIRS SIGNED-RANKS TEST

STATISTICAL TECHNIQUE IN REVIEW

The **Wilcoxon matched-pairs signed-ranks test** is a nonparametric test conducted to examine differences or changes that occur between the first and second observation, such as pretest or posttest measures and matched pairs. This nonparametric test is powerful in the sense that it not only examines the direction of the change, but also the degree of the change. The Wilcoxon test requires a calculation of a difference score for each pair. The greater the amount of change, the more weight the pair is given. When no change occurs, the pair is omitted and the sample size is decreased. Thus, the Wilcoxon matched-pairs signed-ranks test is a strong analysis technique used to examine differences with ordinal level data for related or matched groups. If the result is greater than or equal to ($\geq$) the value in the table, a significant difference exists. If values are statistically significant, the null hypothesis is rejected (Burns & Grove 2005).

RESEARCH ARTICLE

Source: Francis, C. C., Bope, A. A., MaWhinney, S., Czajka-Narins, D., & Alford, B. B. (1999). Body composition, dietary intake, and energy expenditure in nonobese, prepubertal children of obese and nonobese biological mothers. *Journal of the American Dietetic Association, 99*(1), 58–65.

Introduction

According to Francis et al. (1999), research examining nonobese children and their predisposition to obesity is lacking. Therefore, in an effort to determine the differences among body composition, dietary intake, and energy expenditure, the researchers examined height, weight, body mass index (BMI), abdominal fat, body fat, and fat-free mass among prepubertal children of obese and nonobese mothers. This cross-sectional comparison study included a sample of 24 children in 12 pairs, including 5 pairs of boys and 7 pairs of girls matched for age, gender, and weight. Because the subjects were matched for age and weight, there were no Wilcoxon values reported for either of these variables. Subjects' mothers were recruited from flyers and local newspaper, television, and radio advertisements. Due to the small sample size, the Wilcoxon signed-ranks test was chosen to determine any differences among the two groups of children.

Relevant Study Results

"All children and their parents were white. The children in each group were matched for age, gender, and weight" (Francis et al., 1999, p. 62). In Table 1, the researchers presented the demographic and anthropometric characteristics of the sample, which included children of nonobese mothers and children of obese mothers. The differences between the pairs was examined using a Wilcoxon matched-pairs signed-ranks test with the *p* values identified in the last column of Table 1. The level of significance for the study was set at $\alpha = 0.05$. "The significantly higher percentage of abdominal fat and lower fat-free mass in children of obese mothers may contribute to obesity onset. Use of a dual-energy x-ray absorptiometry as a screening tool for nonobese, prepubertal children with an obese parent will help to identify those at risk. Education and lifestyle changes can then be implemented to help prevent the onset of obesity" (Francis et al., 1999, p. 58).

TABLE 1 ■ Demographic and Anthropometric Characteristics of Children of Nonobese and Obese Mothers

	CHILDREN OF NONOBESE MOTHERS[a]			CHILDREN OF OBESE MOTHERS[a]			MEDIAN DIFFERENCE BETWEEN PAIRS			
Variable	Median	Minimum	Maximum	Median	Minimum	Maximum	Median	Minimum	Maximum	*p*[b]
AGE										
Total group	8.5	6	10.5	8.3	6.5	10.5	0.25	−0.5	0.5	
Boys	7.5	7	10.5	7	6.5	10.5				
Girls	8.5	6	10	8.5	6.5	9.5				
WEIGHT (KG)										
Total group	26.4	18.1	38.2	25.6	18.4	39.2	0.55	−3.5	3.7	
Boys	26.1	22.6	38.2	23.4	21.9	39.2				
Girls	26.6	18.1	35.7	27.2	18.4	39.2				
HEIGHT (CM)										
Total group	131.3	112.6	145.5	129.6	115.2	145.4	−0.25	−2.9	10.3	0.93
Boys	129.5	122.2	144.5	125.6	121	142.2				
Girls	133.2	112.6	145.5	135.2	115.2	145.5				
BODY MASS INDEX										
Total group	15.9	13.8	18.3	15.5	13.9	19.4	0.19	−1.9	1.4	0.97
Boys	16.2	15.1	18.3	15.3	14.1	19.4				
Girls	15.3	13.8	16.9	15.9	13.9	18.5				
ABDOMINAL FAT (%)										
Total group	10.9	6.2	20.9	12.9	8	32.9	−3.15	−17.7	0	0.001
Boys	12.3	6.2	20.9	13.3	10.8	24.5				
Girls	9.7	7.4	15.2	12.7	8	32.9				
BODY FAT (%)										
Total group	15.3	11.5	26.2	18.3	12.2	31.6	−2	−11.4	5.4	0.06
Boys	18.5	11.5	26.2	17.8	13.9	24.9				
Girls	14.3	12	20.2	18.8	12.2	31.6				
FREE-FAT MASS (kg)										
Total group	22.1	14.8	28	20.2	14.5	28.8	1.19	−1.3	4.8	0.04
Boys	22.3	18.1	27.5	18.7	16.9	28.8				
Girls	22	14.8	28	21.7	14.5	26				

[a] Total group (*n* = 12 pairs) listed first for each characteristic; boys: *n* = 5 pairs; girls: *n* = 7 pairs
[b] Wilcoxon signed-ranks test

Francis, C. C., Bope, A. A., MaWhinney, S., Czajka-Narins, D., & Alford, B. B. (1999). Body composition, dietary intake, and energy expenditure in nonobese, prepubertal children of obese and nonobese biological mothers. *Journal of the American Dietetic Association, 99*(1), p. 59.

■ STUDY QUESTIONS

1. What was the sample size for this study? How many subjects were in the male and female groups?

2. What was the median value for Weight (kg): Boys for Children of nonobese mothers? What was the median value for Weight (kg): Boys for Children of obese mothers? In your own opinion, are these results expected or unexpected? Provide a rationale for your answer.

3. What was the p value for the Wilcoxon matched-pairs signed-ranks test for Height (cm): Total group? What does this p value indicate?

4. According to Francis et al. (1999), the level of statistical significance for this study was set at 0.05 or $\alpha = 0.05$. What does α mean?

5. What was the Wilcoxon matched-pairs signed-ranks test p value for Fat-free mass (kg): Total group? Was the p value statistically significant? Provide a rationale for your answer.

6. Which variable had a greater statistically significant difference, Body fat (%): Total group or Fat-free mass (kg): Total group?

7. For the variable Body fat (%): Total group, should the null hypothesis be accepted or rejected? Provide a rationale for your answer.

8. For the variable Fat-free mass (kg): Total group, should the null hypothesis be accepted or rejected? Provide a rationale for your answer.

9. The average body mass index (BMI) for the fathers of both groups, fathers of children of nonobese mothers and fathers of children of obese mothers, exceeded 25. In fact, 8 fathers, 4 from each group, reported a BMI greater than 30. The authors report a healthy BMI to be less than 25. In reviewing Table 1, how might this information affect the results of this study?

■ ANSWERS TO STUDY QUESTIONS

1. The sample size was 12 matched pairs consisting of 24 children, 5 male pairs ($n = 5$ pairs) and 7 female pairs ($n = 7$), as indicated in Table 1 and the "Introduction" to the study.

2. The median Weight (kg): Boys for Children of nonobese mothers was 26.1 kg. The median Weight (kg): Boys for Children of obese mothers was 23.4 kg. These medians are unexpected since it is anticipated that children of obese mothers would weigh more than children of nonobese mothers. This difference in weight is not significantly different for the two groups.

3. In Table 1, the p value for the Wilcoxon signed-ranks test Height (cm): Total group is $p = .93$. The p value is nonsignificant since it is greater than $\alpha = 0.05$. Thus, no statistically significant difference exists between the two groups for height, and the null hypothesis was accepted.

4. According to Burns and Grove (2005), α is a symbol for the level of significance that is set prior to the conduct of a study and indicates at what level study results become statistically significant. For this study $\alpha = 0.05$, which means that any p values ≤ 0.05 will be statistically significant results and the null hypothesis will be rejected.

5. The Wilcoxon matched-pairs signed-ranks test p value for Fat-free mass (kg): Total group was $p = 0.04$, meaning Fat-free mass (kg) was significantly greater in the children of nonobese mothers when compared with the children of obese mothers. The value for statistical significance for this study was set at $\alpha = 0.05$. Thus, the results for Fat-free mass (kg): Total group is statistically significant since it is < 0.05 with $p = 0.04$.

6. Fat-free mass (kg): Total group has a greater statistically significant value because it is reported significant at $p = 0.04$. Whereas Body fat (%): Total group is reported to have a value of $p = 0.06$ and is not statistically significant since this p value is greater than $\alpha = 0.05$. In this study, Fat-free mass (kg) is statistically significant for the two groups, but Body fat (%) is not.

7. The null hypothesis for Body fat (%): Total group should be accepted. Body fat (%): Total group is not reported as statistically significant with $p = 0.06$, which is greater than $\alpha = 0.05$. Thus, the null hypothesis is accepted when no significant difference is found.

8. The null hypothesis for Fat-free mass (kg): Total group should be rejected. Fat-free mass (kg): Total group is reported statistically significant at $p = 0.04$, which is less than $\alpha = 0.05$. Thus, the null hypothesis is rejected when statistical significance is found.

9. Answers may vary. Research has shown a connection between obese parents and their children. For example, children of obese parents are more likely to become obese themselves. If a study is examining body composition in nonobese and obese mothers, and how mothers' weight affects their children, the paternal weight cannot be ignored, as it might be just as likely to affect the child due to lifestyle and genetics. Without controlling for the father's weight, how can the researcher contribute the affects of parental obesity solely to one parent? Additional research in this area is needed.

■ EXERCISE 44   Questions to be Graded

1. What was the median value for Body mass index: Total group for children of nonobese mothers? What was the median value for Body mass index: Total group for children of obese mothers? Are these results unexpected?

2. What was the Wilcoxon matched-pairs signed-ranks test p value for Abdominal fat (%): Total group? Was the value statistically significant, and if so, at what level?

3. Which variable had a greater statistically significant difference, Abdominal fat (%): Total group or Fat-free mass (kg): Total group? Provide a rationale for your answer.

4. How many null hypotheses were accepted in this study? How many null hypotheses were rejected? Provide rationales for your answers. Remember that the groups were matched on age and weight and were not examined for differences for these two variables.

5. State the null hypothesis for Abdominal fat (%): Total group. Should this hypothesis be accepted or rejected? Provide a rationale for your answer.

6. What were the minimum and maximum values for Abdominal fat (%): Total group for children of nonobese mothers? Name the type and purpose of this analysis technique. Why were the values for Total group and Boys the same?

7. Why did the authors choose to use a Wilcoxon matched-pairs signed-ranks test? Why are the variables of age and weight lacking a Wilcoxon test value?

8. Was there a control group in this study? What type of study is this? Provide a rationale for your answer.

9. In your own opinion, were the results for Abdominal fat (%), Fat-free mass (kg), Body fat (%), and Body mass index of this study what you expected?

10. All of the participants in this study were Caucasian. How does this characteristic affect the ability to generalize the results to other populations? Provide a rationale for your answer.

EXAMINING SENSITIVITY AND SPECIFICITY OF DIAGNOSTIC AND SCREENING TESTS

STATISTICAL TECHNIQUE IN REVIEW

What laboratory or imaging study do we order to help us screen for or diagnose a disease? When we order a test, are the results valid or accurate? The **accuracy of a screening test** or a test used to confirm a diagnosis is evaluated in terms of its ability to correctly assess the presence or absence of a disease or condition as compared to a gold standard. If the test is positive, what is the probability that the disease is present? If the test is negative, what is the probability that the disease is not present? When we talk to the patient about the results of their tests, how sure are we that they do or do not have the disease? **Sensitivity** and **specificity** are the terms used to describe the accuracy of a screening test. There are four possible outcomes of a screening test for a disease: (1) **true positive**, which is an accurate identification of the presence of a disease, (2) **false positive**, which indicates a disease is present when it is not, (3) **true negative**, which indicates accurately that a disease is not present, or (4) **false negative**, which indicates that a disease is not present when it is. A 2 × 2 contingency table is helpful in visualizing sensitivity and specificity and their four outcomes (Table 45-1).

Sensitivity = Probability of disease = $a/(a+c)$ = True positive rate

Specificity = Probability of no disease = $d/(b+d)$ = True negative rate

Sensitivity is the proportion of patients with the disease who have a positive test result or true positive.

Ways to refer to the test:

- **Highly sensitive test** is very good at identifying the diseased patient.
- If a test is highly sensitive, it has a low percentage of false negatives.
- **Low sensitivity test** is limited in identifying the patient with a disease.
- If a test has low sensitivity, it has a high percentage of false negatives.
- Therefore, if a sensitive test has negative results, the patient is less likely to have the disease.
- Use the acronym SnNout, which is read as: High sensitivity (Sn), test is negative (N), rules the disease out (out).

TABLE 45-1 ■ Results of Sensitivity and Specificity of Screening Tests

	Disease Present	Disease Not Present
Positive test	a (true positive)	b (false positive)
Negative test	c (false negative)	d (true negative)

a = The number of people who have the disease and the test is positive (true positive)
b = The number of people who do not have the disease and the test is positive (false positive)
c = The number of people who have the disease and the test is negative (false negative)
d = The number of people who do not have the disease and the test is negative (true negative)

Specificity is the proportion of patients without the disease who have a negative test result or true negative.

- **Highly specific test** is very good at identifying the patients without a disease.
- If a test is very specific, it has a low percentage of false positives.
- **Low specificity test** is limited in identifying patients without disease.
- If a test has low specificity, it has a high percentage of false positives.
- Therefore, if a specific test has positive results, the patient is more likely to have the disease.
- Use the acronym SpPin, which is read as: High specificity (Sp), test is positive (P), rules the disease in (in).

RESEARCH ARTICLE

Source: Porter, S. C., Fleisher, G. R., Kohane, I. S., & Mandl, K. D. (2003). The value of parental report for diagnosis and management of dehydration in the emergency department. *Annals of Emergency Medicine, 41*(2), 196–205.

Introduction

Porter et al. (2003) conducted a prospective observational study to assess the predictive value of parents reporting the medical history and physical signs of dehydration in their children. Their study included 132 parent-child dyads. The primary outcome was percentage of dehydration, and the secondary outcomes were clinically important acidosis and hospital admission. They also compared the reports of physical signs of dehydration made by the parents and the nurse. Their study results indicated that parents' report of physical symptoms and history had a higher sensitivity (range 73% to 100%) than specificity (range 0% to 49%) for predicting dehydration of 5% or greater in their child (Porter et al., 2003, p. 196).

Relevant Study Results

The researchers presented the results of their study in table format. Table 3 displays the results from the parents' reported history, and Table 4 displays the comparison of the diagnostic value of the parents' and nurses' physical assessment of the clinically important signs of dehydration.

TABLE 3 ■ Value of Parent-Reported History for Prediction of Clinically Important Dehydration

Historical Element (Total No. of Parents = 132)	% Sensitivity (95% CI)	% Specificity (95% CI)
Decreased oral intake	100 (75–100)	18 (8–28)
Decreased urine output	100 (75–100)	26 (15–37)
History of any vomiting during illness	100 (75–100)	3 (0–7)
History of vomiting in past 12 hours	73 (37–92)	6 (0–12)
History of any diarrhea during illness	91 (63–99)	28 (17–39)
History of diarrhea in past 12 hours	82 (50–97)	38 (26–50)
Contact with PCP by telephone (*n* = 131)	91 (63–99)	23 (12–34)
Contact with PCP in office (*n* = 131)	100 (75–100)	49 (36–62)
Previous trial of clear liquids (*n* = 131)	100 (75–100)	22 (12–32)

Porter, S. C., Fleisher, G. R., Kohane, I. S., & Mandl, K. D. (2003). The value of parental report for diagnosis and management of dehydration in the emergency department. *Annals of Emergency Medicine, 41*(2), p. 201.

TABLE 4 ■ Diagnostic Value of Parents and Nurses' Report of Physical Signs for Clinically Important Dehydration*

Physical Sign (No. of Parents/No. of Nurses)	% SENSITIVITY		% SPECIFICITY	
	Parent (95% CI)	Nurse (95% CI)	Parent (95% CI)	Nurse (95% CI)
Ill appearance (71/68)	91 (63–99)	90 (60–99)	17 (7–26)	33 (21–45)
Sunken fontanelle† (13/11)	0 (0–84)	100 (2–100)	82 (48–98)	90 (56–100)
Sunken eyes (71/68)	64 (33–86)	70 (38–91)	37 (15–58)	59 (47–72)
Decreased tears‡ (67/42)	91 (63–99)	100 (33–100)	25 (14–36)	33 (21–45)
Dry mouth (71/68)	64 (33–86)	100 (73–100)	42 (35–48)	49 (36–62)
Weak cry§ (71/41)	54 (25–80)	25 (1–75)	27 (16–38)	78 (65–92)
Cool extremities (71/68)	27 (8–63)	10 (1–40)	73 (62–84)	93 (87–100)

* The total number of patients for this outcome equals 71. Three patients from the subset of 71 did not have nursing assessments for physical signs completed.
† Subset of 32 infants < 9 months of age with only 2 cases of significant dehydration.
‡ Parents and nurses could answer "no opportunity to observe," resulting in missing data for parents (4 patients) and nurses (26 patients).
§ Nurses could answer "no opportunity to observe," resulting in missing data (27 patients).
Porter, S. C., Fleisher, G. R., Kohane, I. S., & Mandl, K. D. (2003). The value of parental report for diagnosis and management of dehydration in the emergency department. *Annals of Emergency Medicine, 41*(2), p. 202.

■ STUDY QUESTIONS

1. Discuss the sensitivity of a screening test and its importance in diagnosing a disease.

2. Discuss the specificity of a screening test and its importance in diagnosing a disease.

3. In Table 3, identify the signs of dehydration (the screening tests) reported by the parents that are 100% sensitive.

4. In Table 3, identify the signs of dehydration reported by the parents that are 100% specific.

5. In Table 3, are the signs of dehydration reported by the parents more sensitive or more specific? Provide a rationale for your answer.

6. Based on your answer to Question 5, are the signs of dehydration reported by the parents more likely to be false positives, true positives, false negatives, or true negatives? Provide a rationale for your answer.

7. Based on the specificity (true negative, i.e., when the test is negative and the disease is not present) of Decreased oral intake reported in Table 3, if parents report that their child does have Decreased oral intake, what percentage of the time will that report be a false positive?

8. Using the information in Table 3, fill in the table below.

SCREENING TEST	DISEASE	
	Dehydration	
Contact with PCP by Telephone	Yes	No
Yes	True positive (a) (91%)	False positive (b) (__%)
No	False negative (c) (9%)	True negative (d) (23%)
	100%	100%
	a/(a+c) = sensitivity = true positives	*d/(d+b) = specificity = true negatives*

9. Using the information in Table 3, fill in the table below.

SCREENING TEST	DISEASE	
	Dehydration	
History of Vomiting in past 12 Hours	Yes	No
Yes	True positive (a) (73%)	False positive (b) (__%)
No	False negative (c) (__%)	True negative (d) (6%)
	100%	100%
	a/(a+c) = sensitivity = true positives	*d/(d+b) = specificity = true negatives*

ANSWERS TO STUDY QUESTIONS

1. Sensitivity of a test indicates the portion of patients who have the disease and have positive test results. The higher the sensitivity of a screening test, the more likely the test is to be positive when a person has a disease, that is, true positive.

2. Specificity of a test indicates the proportion of the patients who do not have a disease and have negative test results. The higher the specificity of a screening test, the more likely the test is to be negative when a person does not a disease, that is, true negative. A test that is both sensitive and specific identifies the patients with disease and rules out those that do not have disease.

3. The 100% sensitivity signs of dehydration indicating that there is 100% consistency between the positive test for the signs of dehydration and actually having the disease of dehydration include:
   a. Decreased oral intake 100% true positives (This sign is always present when the patient has dehydration.)
   b. Decreased urine output 100% true positives
   c. History of any vomiting during illness 100% true positives
   d. Contact with PCP in office 100% true positives
   e. Previous trial of clear liquids 100% true positives

4. None of the specificity values are 100% true negatives. The highest specificity value was 49% for the Contact with PCP in Office.

5. The screening tests for dehydration in Table 3 are more sensitive than specific. The dehydration signs have much higher percentages for sensitivity than specificity. All of the dehydration signs reported by the parents are sensitive at 73% to 100%, and they are specific at only 0% to 49%.

6. The dehydration signs are more likely to be true positives (test identifies a disease when it is present) since they have high sensitivity mean percentages of 73% to 100%. Five of the dehydration signs have 100% sensitivity or true positives and 0% false negatives.

7. 82% is the false positive. Calculation: False Positive = 100% – mean % specificity

$$\text{False positive} = 100\% - 18\% = 82\%$$

8.

SCREENING TEST	DISEASE	
	Dehydration	
Contact with PCP by Telephone	Yes	No
Yes	True positive (a) (91%)	False positive (b) (77%)
No	False negative (c) (9%)	True negative (d) (23%)
	100%	100%
	a/(a+c) = sensitivity = true positives	*d/(d+b) = specificity = true negatives*

9.

SCREENING TEST	DISEASE	
	Dehydration	
History of vomiting in past 12 hours	Yes	No
Yes	True positive (a) (73%)	False positive (b) (94%)
No	False negative (c) (27%)	True negative (d) (6%)
	100%	100%
	a/(a+c) = sensitivity = true positives	*d/(d+b) = specificity = true negatives*

■ EXERCISE 45   Questions to be Graded

1. In Table 4, which two physical signs used by the parents to assess dehydration were the most sensitive? Provide a rationale for your answer.

2. In Table 4, which two physical signs used by the parents to assess dehydration were the most specific? Discuss the meaning of the specificity of these two physical signs.

3. In Table 4, for which physical signs of dehydration did the nurses have more true positives than the parents?

4. In Table 4, which physical signs of dehydration did the nurses have more true negatives than the parents?

5. In Table 4, what is the percentage of false negatives for dehydration if the parents reported Decreased tears? Please provide your calculations.

6. What does it mean if a screening test is 100% sensitive, as Decreased tears was when reported by nurses?

7. What is your interpretation of the specificity of Ill appearance as an indicator for clinical dehydration?

8. Were the nurses or the parents more sensitive and specific in the reporting of the physical signs of dehydration? Was this an expected finding?

9. Fill in the table below using the results from Table 4.

SCREENING TEST	DISEASE	
	Dehydration	
Sunken Eyes	Yes	No
Yes	True positive (a) (70%)	False positive (b) (__%)
No	False negative (c) (__%)	True negative (d) (59%)
	100%	100%
	a/(a+c) = sensitivity = true positives	d/(d+b) = specificity = true negatives

10. Fill in the table below using the results from Table 4.

SCREENING TEST	DISEASE	
	Dehydration	
Weak Cry Reported	Yes	No
Yes	True positive (a) (25%)	False positive (b) (__%)
No	False negative (c) (__%)	True negative (d) (78%)
	100%	100%
	a/(a+c) = sensitivity = true positives	d/(d+b) = specificity = true negatives

■ BONUS QUESTION

Colonoscopy is 95% sensitive and 90% specific in the detection and prevention of colon cancer, and a sigmoidoscopy is 78% sensitive and 70% specific. Which test would you select for your patient who is 50 years of age and has no family history of colon cancer? Provide a rationale for your answer.

REFERENCES

Burns, N., & Grove, S. K. (2005). *The practice of nursing research: Conduct, critique, and utilization,* ed 5, St. Louis, Saunders.

Burns, N., & Grove, S. K. (2007). *Understanding nursing research: Building an evidence-based practice,* ed 4, St. Louis, Saunders.

Munro, B. H. (2001). *Statistical methods for health care research,* ed 4, Philadelphia: Lippincott, Williams & Wilkins.

INDEX